212-570-8568

LAUNCHING THE ANTIBIOTIC ERA

Personal Accounts of the
Discovery and Use
of the First Antibiotics

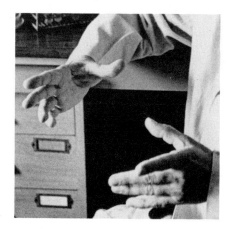

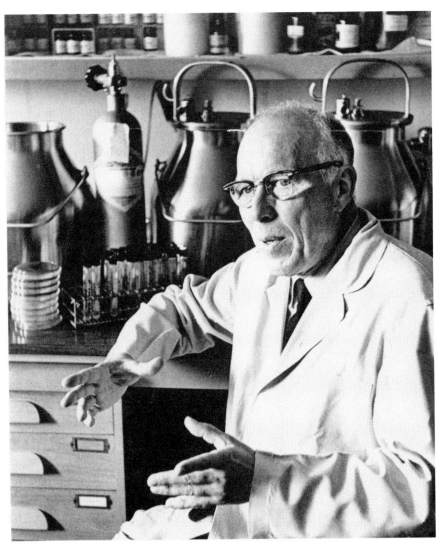

René Dubos, November 1964. Courtesy of Medical World News Collection at Harris County Medical Archive, Houston, Texas. Photo: Roy Stevens.

LAUNCHING THE ANTIBIOTIC ERA

Personal Accounts of the
Discovery and Use
of the First Antibiotics

Edited by
CAROL L. MOBERG
ZANVIL A. COHN

The Rockefeller
University Press
New York · 1990

CONTENTS

PREFACE

This volume represents the proceedings of a symposium held in Caspary Auditorium at The Rockefeller University on October 23, 1989, in commemoration of the fiftieth anniversary of the discovery of gramicidin by René Dubos. Reported in the scientific literature in 1939, gramicidin was the first antibacterial agent to be obtained from natural sources through rational pursuit.

For many, René Dubos is best remembered for his skills as a biographer, philosopher of humankind, and staunch protector of the environment. Yet it was his earlier career as a microbiologist that established his scientific credentials and led to his credibility as a spokesperson for science.

Dubos's discoveries of gramicidin, of an enzyme degrading pneumococcal capsular polysaccharide, of ribonuclease, and of a novel medium for the growth of the tubercle bacillus all stand as exciting milestones in his early career at The Rockefeller Institute for Medical Research. Although Dubos was trained first as an agronomist, then as a journalist, and later as a soil microbiologist, his interests always centered on biomedicine and human well-being. A practicality born of his Gallic background, a Pasteurian influence, and the independence afforded those working at the early Institute all combined to engender a career marked by marvelous versatility and productivity. Few scientists have maintained Dubos's level of intensity and involvement over such a long career.

This fiftieth anniversary also provided the occasion to recall other events leading to the beginning of the antibiotic era and effective antimicrobial therapy. We were fortunate to have with us for this symposium men who were at the forefront of their science. Their personal reminiscences reveal the excitement of a time in which one biological and chemical triumph after another led to a transformation in the therapy of infectious disease.

Their reports reveal more than the bare facts of discovery; they paint a picture of the science and scientists of fifty years ago. Interpersonal relationships, the competitive aspects of research, personal gain, and the role of industry all sound a current note.

Other aspects of the times are also revealed—the important role of The Rockefeller Foundation in supporting young investigators and global research, the opportunities afforded single investigators working in small laboratories, the efficacy of personal involvement at the bedside, and a moral climate that led to patents for the general good. Each aspect of the working investigator and his environment is worthy of reflection in this modern age.

Zanvil A. Cohn
Henry G. Kunkel Professor

and

Carol L. Moberg
Research Associate

The Rockefeller University

Acknowledgments

The publication of this volume was made possible by a gift from the Carl and Lily Pforzheimer Foundation.

Funding for the Launching the Antibiotic Era symposium was provided by The Rockefeller University and by Eli Lilly, Pfizer, Inc., and the Merck Company Foundation.

INTRODUCTION

Science is often thought of as an automatic process. In fact it profits from a richness of styles, personalities, and approaches. Science benefits from accidents of personal history and functions within environments strongly shaped by cultural forces. Histories such as the development of antibiotics—and of René Dubos's role in particular—are valuable because they remind us of science's immense diversity.

My first experience with René Dubos was through *The Bacterial Cell*. It is a book that only Dubos could have written, because he brings into sharp focus what we now take for granted—namely, that bacteria are cells. The book is a lucid and accurate summary of the biology of bacteria known through the mid-1940s. The structures and activities of bacteria, how they relate to problems of virulence, immunity, and chemotherapy, and the phenomena of bacterial variability are all impeccably presented. I know of no other work that had in it the seeds of its own obsolescence, since it inspired so many to pick up on his inspirations and challenges. In doing so, they brought about a rapid displacement of what Dubos said and substantially furthered the march of bacteriology.

The Bacterial Cell is the work from which I can say I learned most of the microbiology I know. The print in my copy is literally read off the pages and the covers are about to fall off. The book appeared in 1945 when I was a medical student working in Francis Ryan's laboratory at Columbia University. I was just beginning to think about whether there was a bacterial genetics, and this work was the launching pad for my own investigations. Within a year, I was able to find evidence that genetic recombination did indeed occur and to find in Dubos a critical review of whether such contingencies could be logically imagined.

In 1954, at the dedication of the Waksman Institute at Rutgers University, I had the occasion to quote Dubos's perspectives on bacteria. In 1945, he wrote

> To the biologist of the 19th century, bacteria appeared as the most primitive expression of cellular organization, the very limit of life. . . . In reality, it appears that it is only their small size and the absence of recognized sexual reproduction which has given the illusion that bacteria are "simple" cells.

Only a year later, he referred to the role of DNA in pneumococcal transformation and the beginning of biochemical genetics. He said

> Bacterial variation passes from the collector's box of the naturalist to the sophisticated atmosphere of the biochemical laboratory. One may wonder whether the geneticist will not arrive too late to introduce his jargon into bacteriology.

Here was one of the very few insights where Dubos was wrong, as the science of bacterial genetics soon came into its own.

Dubos was far ahead of the times in so many ways that to this day we cannot quite catch up with him. He was one of the first hard scientists I encountered who had a sense of the need for a humanistic approach to the limits of science and to the consequences of scientific innovation. Consider, for example, all that is conveyed by Dubos's philosophy in his phrase "mirage of health." We may not be willing to go as far as he did to puncture the illusions about what science can do. However, we needed his efforts to broaden our perspectives, which were often too narrow until he touched our lives so poignantly.

The Rockefeller University is proud to celebrate the fiftieth anniversary of René Dubos's discovery of gramicidin and his role in launching the antibiotic era. The personal recollections that follow present yet another phase of his extraordinary personality and pioneering activities.

Joshua Lederberg
President, 1978–1990
The Rockefeller University

FROM MICROBES TO MEDICINE: GRAMICIDIN, RENÉ DUBOS, AND THE ROCKEFELLER

Rollin D. Hotchkiss

The media have been reminding us that fifty years ago our allies and increasingly this country began a struggle to neutralize the evil efforts of mean-spirited and selfishly ambitious men. Even though that task remains unfinished, it is a great pleasure to recall that there was another beginning at that same time which illustrates the widespread good that can come from healthy spirits engaged in worthy adventures. I have been asked to tell you something about the part we at The Rockefeller Institute were privileged to play in early antibiotics development fifty years ago.

I shall write principally about René Dubos, my chief and associate for many years, and our joint work on the tyrothricin he discovered. I also wish to recall work of his teacher, Selman Waksman of Rutgers University. It is also my hope to conjoin the distinguished authors who follow me, with a few words about penicillin.

René Dubos came to The Rockefeller Institute Hospital in 1927 to test his conviction expressed to Oswald T. Avery that natural soils contain microbes able to attack and break down such refractory substances as the type III polysaccharide of pneumococcus. Soon achieving this goal, he had continued with other fruitful

Professor Emeritus, The Rockefeller University. Joined the Avery laboratory in 1935 at age 24. Worked with René Dubos on the identification, purification, and crystallization of gramicidin. Later he made pioneering contributions to DNA research.

experimental studies on the pneumococcus—all more of a biochemical or biological, rather than medical, nature. In 1939 he announced the discovery of what was probably the first antibacterial principle that resulted from a deliberate, somewhat systematic search for antagonistic principles among soil microorganisms.

The Avery lab in 1936 had the concept of a sort of master antigen—made up of protein, carbohydrate, and, according to Dubos, RNA—which was deemed to be the essential skeleton of the pneumococcus and other gram-positive bacteria. Sure that this structure does not survive after it falls into the soil, Dubos began in 1937 a sort of extracurricular experiment. At intervals, he "fed" a large sample of mixed soils with suspensions of living gram-positive bacteria, reasoning that some soil organism would grow there by breaking down the cells he supplied it. At the outset, he was looking for a cell-destroying rather than a growth-preventing agent. In four 1939 reports (1–3) he described an antagonistic strain of bacteria he obtained, and the production from it of an alcohol-soluble principle, to which we later gave the name tyrothricin. It showed the ability to promote the lysis or disintegration of virtually every gram-positive bacterial species tested—and, besides this bacteriolytic activity, it had a powerful growth-inhibitory effect that could also be demonstrated as a protective effect against infections in the animal body.

This is how the first deliberately sought antibiotic was discovered—based on the supremely simple working hypothesis that soil as a self-purifying environment could supply an agent to destroy disease-causing bacteria.

We must pause to consider briefly the status of chemotherapy of bacterial diseases at that time. In 1940, it seemed a prime goal to defeat the gram-positive bacteria—the agents of such major scourges as pneumonia, diphtheria, scarlet fever, anthrax, and all sorts of streptococcal or staphylococcal infections, etc. Some could be moderated with the use of a specific immuneserum or antibody. But as I have noted elsewhere (4), the chemotherapeutic agents available in the 1930s were almost all based upon poisonous principles—arsenic, mercury, phenols, fatty acids, complex basic dyes, etc.—which were rendered less broadly poisonous to animal and host tissue by artful chemical group substitution or modification. Guided by Paul Ehrlich's concept of the "magic bullet," one usually started with such a lethal-bullet principle—which an enterprising chemical industry then tried to "detoxify" into an arsphenamine or salvarsan, a mercurochrome, cresol, hexylresorcinol, or a dye molecule that would target the trypanosomes. These were the challenges and attitudes, as I well knew, that motivated and channeled a generation of organic chemists—my classmates and contemporaries.

But sulfanilamide had just appeared on this horizon; new in 1937, its magic was beginning to be appreciated, though we had not yet been shown that it was a chemically modified vitamin rather than a modified poison. The stage was set for kinder, gentler drugs and at first it seemed that Dubos's agent could be one. Something elaborated by living bacteria was showing the specificity we dreamed of: toxicity for one whole class of cells, but little or none for itself and some others. Quite on my own, in the middle of 1939 I volunteered to help Dubos purify the bacterial extract he had produced. My adventure did not have the sanction or encouragement of my administrative superiors—not until I had made some progress and we were deeper into World War II. But I shall always be grateful to The Rockefeller Institute for permitting us to initiate our own war research project.

We contrived to commandeer some lab help and some large equipment for a summer of growing gallons of the soil organism *Bacillus brevis* and preparing the raw material Dubos had isolated. The crude brownish material was practically incompatible with water and, under organic solvents, congealed into a sticky mass as unpleasant as so much uncouth earwax. But it was powerful wax all right. Its amber alcohol solutions could be finessed into an acceptable suspension in water, and at great dilutions it would powerfully block bacterial growth, both in the test tube and in the peritoneal cavity of an infected mouse. Starting with some half a pound of the material, I set out that fall to find the nature of its powers.

Needing to manipulate a good many liters of different hot organic solvents, including ether, I soon attracted the attention of other colleagues. I was banished to the Power House roof for fear that I would set fire to our Hospital patients, rather than simply reduce their fevers. Now the admirable traditions of The Rockefeller Institute administration to ease the toil of honest research came to our aid. Soon I was granted my first technical assistant, and we were given keys to unlock and work in the lavish mouse dormitory and surgery which Alexis Carrel had built and abandoned when he moved to Europe. There I was enabled to set up some explosion-proof, safe electrical equipment and bring in other supplies.

I tried out hundreds of differential solubility tests with the brown waxes. A manipulation that appeared promising on a small pilot sample was repeated, perhaps slightly differently, with a larger batch. Figure 1 shows two pages (out of seventeen similar ones in my notebooks) which give a picture (details are not important) of the general trial-and-error nature of the process. Gradually it became clear that two kinds of products were present: one rather more soluble than the other in alcohol containing a high proportion of ether. Then began an intense side-by-side collaboration as Dubos and I followed this fractionation in biological assays. At many of my innumerable little steps, I'd make up a dilute solution of my fraction and we'd set up together test tube and mouse assays to see where matters stood. Arriving at the lab each day a good hour before I did, René would absorb the information the night had brought. From my end, I could usually tell him

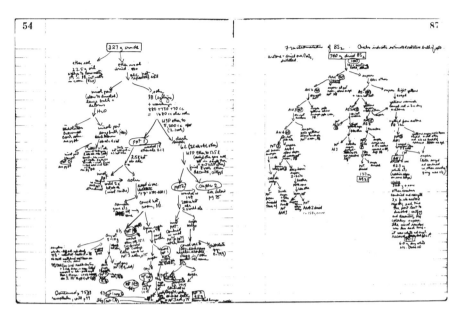

Figure 1. Reproduction of two pages from author's notebook illustrating the general nature and flow of early pilot experiments on fractionation of tyrothricin. Each arrow indicates a small or large sample being manipulated in various pure or mixed organic solvents.

whether the mice had looked feverish or nonchalant—noncalorific—at midnight. With all night to think about it, my cautious evaluations had usually caught up to his instant insights of the next day, so we quickly made our conclusions. They pointed us toward signs that I was separating a bacteriolytic, and hemolytic, agent from a milder agent which on the other hand was far more powerful in combatting the infections in mice. Before long I had them as pure white crystals: first, the roughneck lysin (we later named this one tyrocidine hydrochloride), and then, on November 4, 1939, the gentle protector, which we named gramicidin.

The fractionation scheme as eventually published (5, 6; fig. 2) took all of the romance out of the process; in fact it presents only the principle of purification, not a recipe or prescription for processing. A small industry started up based on these steps and for a time prepared multigram quantities of our products.

The name *tyrothricin* for the crude material came from a probable relation to Tyrothrix bacteria (threads from cheese). Hence also tyrocidine, for a "killer from cheese." For our subtle bacterial inhibitor, we chose the term *gramicidin*, not to signify killing Hans Christian Gram, but because it killed the gram-positive bacteria he taught us how to stain and recognize. Figure 3 shows photomicrographs of tyrocidine and gramicidin.

Considerable excitement had been aroused in biochemical and biomedical colleagues and in industry. René Dubos and I each gave papers at a 1939 Christmastime bacteriology meeting in New Haven. We had been designing chemotherapeutic assays of my crystalline substances, but I had not yet found out much about their composition. Hoping to escape premature intense questioning, I created something of a stir by quietly announcing at the outset of my talk that questions about the chemistry "would only be embarrassing to the speaker and disappointing to the questioner"! However, René could tell them that one microgram of gramicidin would protect mice from thousands of otherwise fatal doses of pneumococcus. And the onlookers liked the curious characteristic rounded cigar- or boat-shape of the gramicidin crystals. Since at that time the German attack boat, the *Graf Spee,* had eluded the British Navy after creating notorious damage to North Sea shipping, I showed my picture of crystals with the comment "we should all try to locate the *Graf Spee!*" Before the New Year we released, to all drug companies and colleagues who requested it, the special *B. brevis* culture, together with full instructions for making the crude and purified extracts. By February 1940 we had published notes with further details (7).

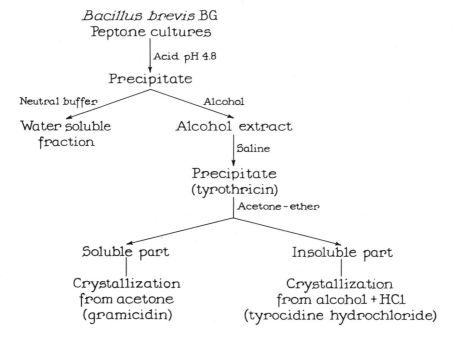

Figure 2.   General description of fractionation scheme for separating raw tyrothricin into fractions yielding tyrocidine-HCl and gramicidin.

We had high hopes that we had a powerful new curative and preventive medicine, and so did the directors of research at The Rockefeller Institute. I recall speculations that our preparations might eventually be added to fresh milk, and beer or other products, to obviate the need for pasteurization. One might ask, in a mercantile world, "What in the world was The Rockefeller Institute doing—in its Hospital!—letting a soil microbiologist and a footloose organic chemist follow their unorthodox dreams?" (Dubos has mused along this line also.) I can only say that the policy of taking such "calculated risks," especially with ideas that come up "from below," still seems to me one of the best features of an enlightened institution for research.

It is best of all when administration follows a program with interest as well as support. The directors asked us to make a patent application, which they hoped would save the potent elixir for the general good, as required by the Rockefeller charter. And so two patent lawyers experienced only in defined chemical compounds began to coach two unworldly experimenters who knew little about their undefined products, and far less about such practical matters as talking bigger in inverse proportion to what they knew. But we skimmed the contents of our notebooks and whipped the cream up into thirty-six hopelessly vague patent

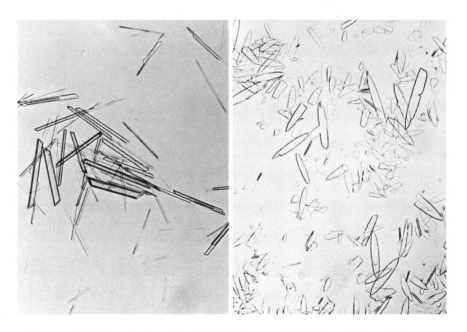

Figure 3. (Left) *Crystals of tyrocidine hydrochloride.* ×320. (Right) *Crystals of gramicidin.* ×225.

claims. When Dubos and I were officially assigning these patent revelations over to the Institute, we pointed optimistically to the clause "in consideration of the sum of one dollar"—what we understood to be a legal minimum to bid one forever hold his peace. At this the Institute's kindly business manager, the towering E. B. Smith, disappeared and then returned, bringing into the room two shiny half dollars, with which he crossed our respective palms—one for each! That has kept me "halfway peaceful" but I've often wished that I had preserved that tangible token of a great institution's pragmatic philanthropy! Our own grand gesture, too, came to little; the patent application was abandoned later on, with the gradual recognition that our substances were toxic and that the mere application moreover had served its purpose of preventing one-sided exploitation.

There followed a partly cooperative, partly competitive period I shall never forget. In a few months such major laboratories as Parke, Davis & Co., Merck, Squibb, Sharpe and Dohme, Lederle, and Lilly had given us courtesy samples of tyrothricin varying from five to one hundred grams, and a few early reports on their crash chemical examination of it. Knowing that these contemporaries and ex-classmates were earning two or three times my salary, I was fascinated to see that even a flock of experts can be astonishingly clumsy when a big corporation demands that they rush to prepare and analyze a material before their hearts and minds are yet involved in it. But in time a few of them did get involved, and set up teams, often of several chemists, to study our substances. At a Federated Societies meeting in 1941, I briefly reported the polypeptide composition of tyrocidine and gramicidin. Halvor Christensen, from Lederle Laboratories (supplier of the generous hundred-gram sample of tyrothricin), came to the meeting with data of his own. Refreshed by late-telephoned lab news that morning, my friend rose to present his "independent observations" as discussion to my little twelve-minute paper! Well, he added some details and confirmations; his crystalline tyrocidine was lower in tryptophan content than mine, so he probably was foreshadowing the later findings of Gregory and Craig (8) and King and Craig (9) that these polypeptides occurred in little families with small differences in amino acid composition. In most points we were in approximate agreement; the same was true of work by another team led by Max Tishler at Merck. Gordon, Martin, and Synge (10) also had a "mixed" tyrocidine, but their introduction of new micromethods brought more precise results, later amplified by the aforementioned work of Craig and co-workers.

A curious confirmation arose from the work of another colleague, J. C. Hoogerheide, at the Biochemical Research Institute in Delaware, on soil cultures that inhibited capsule synthesis in certain bacteria (11). When he saw our first reports he noted similarities; he had in a different but thoroughly professional way come upon the same *Bacillus brevis* system! He quickly confirmed most of our observations, but his director was not satisfied with that. In June 1940, Ellice McDonald published a grandiose Franklin Institute–wide report (12) summarizing these duplicate findings, complete with a picture of the boat-shaped crystals. But he claimed that their material might be different from gramicidin, since it had a nitrogen content one percent higher than we had reported (we were the ones in error: our analyst did not recover all the tryptophan nitrogen). Members of his staff acknowledged the identity in an article two years later (13) that did not even mention the director's confrontational publication.

It became clear that gramicidin could be tolerated by cells much better than tyrocidine, although the latter was less toxic—also less effective—in the presence of serum or proteins. I devised a demonstration suitable for a biochemistry laboratory (6). Fertilized frog eggs were exposed to the agents, and it could easily be seen (fig. 4) that their development was abruptly stopped by tyrocidine, while

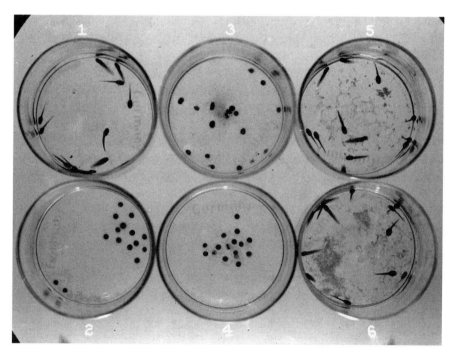

Figure 4. Frog embryos after a six-day exposure to (1) control; (2) 63 μg/ml tyrothricin; (3) 6.5 μg/ml tyrocidine; (4) 38 μg/ml tyrocidine; (5) 63 μg/ml gramicidin; and (6) 310 μg/ml gramicidin. The crude mixture, tyrothricin, and purified tyrocidine derived from it blocked embryonic development at approximately the time of addition; gramicidin had no obvious effect on development (see reference 6).

tadpoles developed and swam unconcernedly amidst the precipitate of excess gramicidin. During the early years of the war, gramicidin was shown to be effective in topical application to localized infections of body cavities, such as otitis, ulcers, and wounds. For a time it saved lives and productivity in herds of cows afflicted with mastitis (14, 15), and almost surely of some people whose successfully treated local infections might otherwise have gone on to septicemic blood poisoning. Had we not gained access to improved sulfa drugs and the superior penicillin, it could well have saved some more; it still finds a place in some antiseptic ointments and creams.

Significant scientific results also came from the work. We found tyrocidine and gramicidin to be small polypeptides, and as forerunners of cyclic peptides and of such antibacterial agents as polymyxin and bacitracin, they had some place in history. We showed that they contained some "unnatural" or D-amino acids (16); that is, inverted versions of the widespread usual components of proteins. This last work was done in collaboration with Fritz Lipmann, who thereby became interested and for some years involved with several aspects of the action and biosynthesis of these polypeptides. He and his co-workers established (17, 18) that these peptides are synthesized independently of the DNA/RNA-coding route, which is probably why they can include D-amino acids and can admit of some variations in sequence.

Gramicidin has a subtle effect upon bacterial metabolism. After I discovered that it (and also dinitrophenol) blocks phosphate incorporation by respiring cells (6), I briefly explored these effects in mammalian systems. Table I provides evidence that gramicidin markedly inhibits inorganic phosphate esterification (a process which stores the metabolic energy) of cell-free extracts of rabbit kidney. This very table was presented in 1944 (19) at a symposium arranged and chaired by Lipmann. A few years later he confirmed and extended some of those findings (20). Unfortunately, I never submitted my own results for publication. Lately gramicidin has been seen as a channel-forming agent which alters permeability of cell membranes. If it plays a similar but less harmful role at home in the cells that make it, it may be of the class now called porins—a member discovered long before the others and before the class was defined.

Tyrocidine is far more aggressive in the way it attacks cell membranes. It is a quite complicated member of a large class indeed: the surface-active agents immediately destructive to bacterial membranes. During my wartime work, I showed that it was more antiseptic than chemotherapeutic. The same was true of a peptide isolated in the Soviet Union by G. F. Gause and attributively designated by him Soviet gramicidin, or gramicidin S, although it proved really to be a sister of tyrocidine instead.

Table I.   Effect of gramicidin on phosphorylation in respiring cell-free extract of rabbit kidney tissue.

Exp. No.	NaF	Gramicidin	Phosphate esterified	Oxygen uptake	μmol P esterified per μmol O₂ uptake
	mg/ml	*µg/ml*	*µg*	*µl*	
1	0.5	—	54	234	0.17
	0.5	53	0	287	0.00
	0	—	0	244	0.00
2	1.0	—	58	295	0.14
	1.0	—	73	378	0.14
	1.0	26	0	380	0.00
	1.0	13	0	366	0.00
3	1.1	—	258	428	0.44
	1.1	—	477	542	0.64
	1.1	55	37	399	0.07

Tissue prepared by method of Kalckar (*Enzymologia*, 1937, 2:47), incubated in Warburg manometer flasks for different periods of time (intervals not given, but indicated by proportional oxygen uptake).

The characteristic of tyrocidine killing, I found, was that in conditions and concentrations at which it kills bacteria, tyrocidine allowed the small molecules inside the cell to leak out (21). Broadening this in my wartime work to a wide array of polar–nonpolar surface-active agents (those substances which have one part water-loving and another water-hating), I showed that all of them (more than thirty of different kinds were tested), used at their respective killing concentrations, produced this drastic membrane damage. It became a very sensitive and, moreover, almost instantaneous test for a large class of antiseptics. Whatever specificity they show appears in the concentration at which they are active for a given cell type or environment. In this light, tyrocidine (and gramicidin S!) is only a curiously complicated soap.

In figure 5 you can see examples of this class represented as they would be oriented at a membrane–water interface. A glance at the variety of structures indicated will suggest how broad was the generalization I was able to make. Here we see in the middle some standard soaps and detergents; at the left, tyrocidine (note the complex array of aromatic and fatty side chains poking down into the lipoid phase); at the right, as we allow higher concentrations of less-active substances, we find that the phenols (basis for the old "phenol coefficient" measure of antisepsis) also are surface active. Finally we have trichloroacetic acid (my own and the biochemist's "standard reagent" for extracting small molecules from bacteria); I want to call attention to the fact that at the enormous concentrations at which trichloroacetic acid is used, it too becomes surface active, being a sort of hybrid composed of chloroform on one end and formic acid on the other!

Partners in Penicillin

Although the literature records a good many reports of bacteria and fungi which inhibited growth of bacteria, these were almost without exception chance observations about cultures already isolated and in hand. Penicillin came to Alexander Fleming a little differently. You will read this magnificent story shortly from Edward Abraham and Norman Heatley, but I would like to say how it influenced us as time went on. Well before 1939, Dubos was an admirer of Fleming's work; he often quoted the work on lysozyme by Fleming—and Abraham—and sometimes the discovery of the penicillin strain in 1929 (22) and the inhibitory extract, which had virtually been shelved since that time. His first paper on *Bacillus brevis* (1) refers to the specific effects of penicillin. So all the more Dubos and I both treasured our recollection of a conference at which, after René had spoken about our antibacterial agent, a person identified as Professor Florey arose to say that Dubos's first reports had helped encourage the Oxford group to reconsider penicillin. It seems that our English colleagues are unable to confirm our belief that the occasion was the International Congress of Microbiology opening in New York almost simultaneously with Hitler's invasion of Poland.

Certainly as our work proceeded, we in turn were being stimulated as we learned of the advances in the penicillin work, and we followed it with growing interest. At times, however, our vision may have been cloudy: I recall an amusing episode at some informal discussion in the 1940s; Dubos was asked to state his view of the prospects for penicillin. He attested its marvels all right, but, aware of the reported lability of the then-crude product, he stated in a rather emphatic manner his opinion that it would not be practical. "It will have to be manufactured in big centers, then refrigerated, shipped, and regularly renewed at local sites— also refrigerated—where it is used. And we just don't have that kind of organization and technology," he concluded. While the listeners were pondering this heavy portent, beside me in the group, my friend the late Mark Adams, of bacteriophage fame, turned to me and chuckled, "Well, they do pretty well handling ice

SURFACE-ACTIVE ANTIBACTERIAL AGENTS

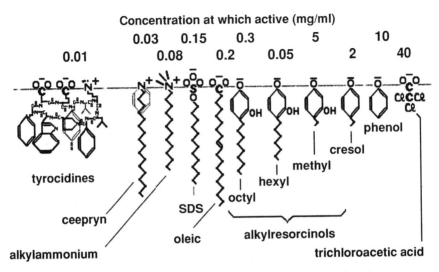

Figure 5. Schematic diagram of various surface-active molecules, as they array themselves at a water–lipid interface (horizontal line). The substances are bactericidal for staphylococci at different concentrations indicated on an approximate numerical scale at top (concentration increasing, activity diminishing, toward the right). The structures are represented in their general shapes; bends and junctions indicate usually the –CH– aliphatic elements. Structures at left indicated in lighter density should be construed as located behind those in darker tone. Soviet "gramicidin S" and tyrocidines A and B are represented by tyrocidine B. (Moderate specificity of various compounds can be revealed in different effective concentrations for different cell species, or at different acidities, etc.)

cream like that!" This quick rejoinder nearly broke me up, but Dubos did not hear Adams's remark until I repeated it to him later—this is the first time I have told it in public. As all may know, purification of penicillin eliminated the concern of its instability!

I visited Fleming's lab on two fortunate occasions. On one (I suppose it was in 1948) he had shown me the famous colony and inhibition zone on a preserved agar plate. After a while he passed me over to an attractive young lady co-worker, with whom I had an enjoyable talk about her, and probably our own, work. As time passed so pleasantly, I asked her if I could take her to dinner that evening. She declined, but countered nicely by taking me to the BBC studios instead and feeding me with packets of macadamia nuts while she read out the news to Greece on the British Overseas News Service. My "date" with this charming lady turned out unexpectedly, and not so long after I was charmed and surprised again to learn that Madame Amalia Voureka had married Fleming.

Professor and Student

At Rutgers it had been Selman Waksman who had taught Dubos about soil micro-organisms and their biochemical versatility. Waksman, an emigré from the Soviet Union in 1911, was a pragmatic and industrious microbiologist, impressed by the opportunities opened up by his emigration and eager to make the most of them and to pass them on to others. In a sense he had never left the soil, and the farmland philosophy that all things good arise from the soil, the people, and hard work. He had emerged as a scholar of the elaborate interactions between biologi-cal and environmental forces in the soil biota—an early ecologist. His visions yearned upward and outward, but his strengths had chiefly been demonstrated in descriptive studies of what went on in the soil and what could be reisolated from it.

Waksman had pondered and tabulated the cooperative and antagonistic effects of various soil organisms upon each other, and Dubos had learned about such effects from him. And Waksman has made it equally clear that in 1939 Dubos's work revealed to him the relatively new idea of experimentally seeking and exploiting such antagonisms. Following Dubos's report, Waksman with Boyd Woodruff (and soon other co-workers) began to search in soil for fresh examples of microorganisms inhibitory to others, and that same year made an arrangement with Merck & Co., Inc. to collaborate for developing this field. He mostly dispensed with the long training enrichment method of Dubos, reducing the search to looking for organisms already there which produced an inhibition zone on solid media. By now the strategy was complete; no longer were they looking for organisms that destroyed and consumed others, but for those that inhibited growth. It was hardly surprising that the media used often ended up with prominent colonies of actinomycetes, his favorite objects of study. Within a few years Waksman had reported scores of inhibitory substances and in 1941 had proposed for them the class name "antibiotics." This term and some of his sub-stances have become household words for us. Table II presents some of the products discovered or worked on in the Waksman laboratory. Over a quarter century, Waksman published 197 papers on antibiotics, many of them original studies, though in time a majority of them were reviews and surveys, for he never relinquished the duty and pleasure of serving as public relations officer for this burgeoning field.

Table II.   Some antibiotics developed in the laboratory of Selman Waksman.

Year	Agent found or tested
1940	(pyocanase); actinomycin
1942	streptothricin; fumagacin; clavacin
1943	*Aspergillus flavus* agent
1944	chaetomin; streptomycin
1945	grisein
1946	*Phycomyces* agent
1947	micromonosporin
1949	neomycin; streptocin
1950	fradicin
1951	rhodomycin; ehrlichin
1952	fungicidin (= nystatin)
1953	candicidin
1954	candidin (= amphotericin)
1956	mycothricins
1957	sulfocidin

Waksman's arrangement with Merck was productive and constructive; a considerable part of his royalties were turned back into research work and one major creation, the Institute for Microbiology, intended as a home for fundamental research under the sponsorship of Rutgers University. Moreover, because of his efforts, Merck was generous in licensing to other manufacturers the greatest achievement of the joint work, streptomycin.

The Personal Contribution

A magic drug is also elusive by the screening route. It was the fourth year, 1944, that brought streptomycin, rewarded with the Nobel Prize for 1952. Table II and Waksman's many papers and patents on antibiotics illustrate for us the great difference in temperament and social function eventually performed by Dubos and his teacher. The student, motivated by a rather romantic philosophical urge, sought large principles working in nature; Waksman, driven by other visions, had perhaps less faith in the strength of ideas, but a naturalist's trust that unique values of special systems will be revealed through systematic hard work and repetition of sometimes boring tasks. So far as I know, Dubos made only one more serious attempt to discover an antibiotic factor: an inhibitor of the tubercle bacillus. I saw some phases of such a search being done together with Gardner Middlebrook. And frequently in lectures and writings he pointed out the weaknesses of purely empirical screening methods. He hardly raised his head to look when I once showed him a paper on the "second one thousand isolations of antibiotics" from soil etc. (as I remember it, an article reported from a screening cooperative).

In public speeches and writings, Dubos gave reasons for his skepticism of the effectiveness of random searches for new antibiotics, and some of his reasoning came from our own experience. He had sought an organism which would "break down" gram-positive bacterial structures, and found such an organism, and from it a lytic antibacterial factor satisfying the specifications of his search. But when purified, the lytic, generally toxic, tyrocidine was not valuable—what was valuable was the serendipitous finding independent of the working hypothesis. Carried along with the tyrocidine was the far more subtle gramicidin—not obviously bacteriolytic. Luckily, gramicidin was saved and therefore we could discover its growth-inhibitory and -protective effects in the animal body against bacterial infections. In fact, the operative screening test brought Dubos something more than it was designed to do, and it was insight and industry which saved that something better! Most people who carried this sort of search forward did not use the prolonged soil enrichment culturing Dubos did (Waksman, as mentioned; see also Stokes and Woodward [23]; Hoogerheide [11]), but I believe Dubos felt that this step might well have increased their chances for an adaptation that would increase useful minor constituents of the soil flora.

Dubos hesitated to adopt the word *antibiotic* itself: in his philosophy a word signifying "against life" was too broad a charge for him since it suggested too many things—general poisoning, acid production, competition for nutrients—besides the rather elegant and specific actions which practical usage nevertheless soon gave the word.

A basic personality trait may also be involved here. I remember Dubos sometimes commenting on the worldly value (a "trick" or gimmick, he considered it) for a scholar of coining a new word and thereby becoming associated with it in science "history." He pointed out that scholars and historians tend to be captivated by word-thinking, and in the literature to search back and to stop when they reach the earliest use (therefore the coiner) of some focal term; e.g., *antibiotics* or *enzymatic adaptation*. But I do not believe he ever deliberately chose this easy route to fame for himself; we had to name our tyrothricin, tyrocidine, and gramicidin, of course, but we did it late, and with misgivings. As I now see it, Dubos's philosophy gave such a "load" of connotations and nuances to any word, that he simply did not enjoy, as many do, choosing a neologism, which is always ambiguous and has to earn the exquisite nicety of a specific new concept. Dubos's creativity found better outlet in phrases and expressions: as in later writings he became known for "the despairing optimist" and the precept "think globally, act locally"—which say so much.

Those aware of the later career of René Dubos will easily recognize the broadening and deepening of the early experimental themes into his writing: ecological interaction; respect for nature and the soil as self-purifying environments if treated with consideration; the possibility of cooperating with natural systems and benefiting from adaptations worked out in their age-old evolution.

We would be overcasting if we fitted these pioneers too nicely into stereotyped character roles in our historical drama: Fleming, the last and most acute of the Ancient Observers; Dubos, the astute Explorer; Waksman, the busy Prospector; Florey and Chain and our British colleagues as the enterprising Developers and Engineers. In truth they all had to be part observer-explorer and engineer, and their intellectual efforts and the patient, innovative work of their hands have opened new doors.

I have a nightmare, in which our world is increasingly given over to people who believe that the profit motive is our only sure guiding principle; that police actions, local and international, are the only true functions of government; that education and research and creativity are best supported by those who have proven themselves in the world of profit making; that persuasive speech is a sure sign of wisdom. When I awaken from this nightmare, as I occasionally do, I rejoice in realizing that—erratically but regularly—there still arise in the world those who build and create. And there can also come the time when someone says, "Enough! I have had enough admiration and profit and prizes! I am not content merely doing well, I will strive to do good!" We may hope that in the general society many will receive such inspiration, as we do today, from such people as Dubos, Waksman, Fleming, Florey, Chain, and from their distinguished associates and fellow spirits who are alive today.

References

1. Dubos, R. J. 1939. Bactericidal effect of an extract of a soil bacillus on Gram-positive cocci. *Proceedings of the Society for Experimental Biology and Medicine.* 40:311.

2. Dubos, R. J. 1939. Studies on a bactericidal agent extracted from a soil bacillus. I. Preparation of the agent. II. Protective effect of the bactericidal agent against experimental pneumococcus infections in mice. *Journal of Experimental Medicine.* 70:1; 70:11.

3. Dubos, R. J., and C. Cattaneo. 1939. Studies on a bactericidal agent extracted from a soil bacillus. III. Preparation and activity of a protein-free fraction. *Journal of Experimental Medicine.* 70:249.

4. Hotchkiss, R. D. 1946. Chemotherapy: applied cytochemistry. In *Currents in Biochemical Research*, edited by D. E. Green, p. 379. New York: Interscience Publishers.

5. Dubos, R. J., and R. D. Hotchkiss. 1942. Origin, nature and properties of gramicidin and tyrocidine. *Transactions & Studies of the College of Physicians of Philadelphia.* 10:11.

6. Hotchkiss, R. D. 1944. Gramicidin, tyrocidine, and tyrothricin. *Advances in Enzymology.* 4:153.

7. Hotchkiss, R. D., and R. J. Dubos. 1940. Fractionation of the bactericidal agent from cultures of a soil bacillus. Chemical properties of bactericidal substances isolated from cultures of a soil bacillus. Bactericidal fractions from an aerobic sporulating bacillus. *Journal of Biological Chemistry.* 132:791; 132:793; 136:803.

8. Gregory, J. D., and L. C. Craig. 1948. Counter-current distribution of gramicidin. *Journal of Biological Chemistry.* 172:839.

9. King, T. P., and L. C. Craig. 1955. The chemistry of tyrocidine. V. The amino acid sequence of tyrocidine B. *Journal of the American Chemical Society.* 77:6627.

10. Gordon, A. H., A. J. P. Martin, and R. L. M. Synge. 1943. The amino-acid composition of gramicidin. The amino-acid composition of tyrocidine. *Biochemical Journal.* 37:86; 37:313.

11. Hoogerheide, J. C. 1940. An agent, isolated from a soil bacillus, which inhibits encapsulation of Friedlander's bacterium and is highly bactericidal for Gram-positive microorganisms. *Journal of the Franklin Institute.* 229:677.

12. McDonald, E. 1940. Further studies on the bactericidal agents obtained from soil bacilli. *Journal of the Franklin Institute.* 229:805.

13. Phillips, R. L. 1942. Development of resistance to staphylococci to natural inhibitory substances. *Journal of the Franklin Institute.* 233:396.

14. Little, R. B., R. J. Dubos, and R. D. Hotchkiss. 1940. Action of gramicidin on streptococci of bovine mastitis. Effect of gramicidin suspended in mineral oil on streptococci of bovine mastitis. *Proceedings of the Society for Experimental Biology and Medicine*. 45:444; 45:462.
15. Little, R. B., R. J. Dubos, and R. D. Hotchkiss. 1941. Gramicidin, novoxil and acriflavine for the treatment of the chronic form of streptococcic mastitis. *Journal of the American Veterinary Medical Association*. 98:189.
16. Lipmann, F., R. D. Hotchkiss, and R. J. Dubos. 1941. The occurrence of D-amino acids in gramicidin and tyrocidine. *Journal of Biological Chemistry*. 141:163.
17. Kleinkauf, H., W. Gevers, and F. Lipmann. 1969. Interrelation between activation and polymerization in gramicidin S biosynthesis. *Proceedings of the National Academy of Sciences of the United States of America*. 62:226.
18. Lee, S., and F. Lipmann. 1977. Isolation of amino acid activating subunit pantetheine-protein complexes: their role in chain elongation in tyrocidine synthesis. *Proceedings of the National Academy of Sciences of the United States of America*. 74:2343.
19. Hotchkiss, R. D. 1945. The mechanism of the bacteriostatic action of gramicidin. Talk before Division of Biological Chemistry, 112th Meeting of the American Chemical Society, New York, 1945. (Abstract 33, p 21B)
20. Loomis, W. F., and F. Lipmann. 1948. Reversible inhibition of the coupling between phosphorylation and oxidation. *Journal of Biological Chemistry*. 173:807.
21. Hotchkiss, R. D. 1946. The nature of the bactericidal action of surface active agents. *Annals of the New York Academy of Sciences*. 46:479.
22. Fleming, A. 1929. On the antibacterial action of cultures of a Penicillium, with special reference to their use in the isolation of *B. influenzae*. *British Journal of Experimental Pathology*. 10:226.
23. Stokes, J. L., and C. E. Woodward, Jr. 1942. The isolation from soil of spore-forming bacteria which produce bactericidal substances. *Journal of Bacteriology*. 43:253.

OXFORD,
HOWARD FLOREY,
AND WORLD WAR II

Edward P. Abraham

It was a great pleasure to me to be invited to this celebration of the fiftieth anniversary of the discovery of gramicidin by René Dubos (with Rollin Hotchkiss) and to visit his scientific home again after thirty years. Forty years ago, in *Antibiotics* (1949), a review of antibiotics from bacteria, Howard Florey and I wrote the following about their research with *Bacillus brevis:* "This work and its continuation had the outstanding merit (in sharp contrast to all previous work) of considering the subject from many points of view—bacteriological, biochemical, biological, and eventually clinical." On the other hand, we could not say what Alexander Fleming had rightly said after learning of the great therapeutic power of penicillin, which was that the fates had been wonderfully kind to him. It seems to me that kinder fates had been deserved by René Dubos, for he would certainly have exploited what they offered him.

 The decision of Florey and Ernst Chain to make a survey of the many antimicrobial substances that had been reported to be produced by microorganisms appears to have emerged from their discussions in 1937–38 and to have preceded the appearance of the paper on gramicidin. These discussions arose from

Professor Emeritus, Sir William Dunn School of Pathology, University of Oxford. Worked with Howard Florey and Ernst Chain to purify and to determine the structure of penicillin. Together with G. G. F. Newton, in 1953, he discovered cephalosporin C, determined its structure, and isolated its nucleus. This led to the introduction of cephalosporins into clinical medicine.

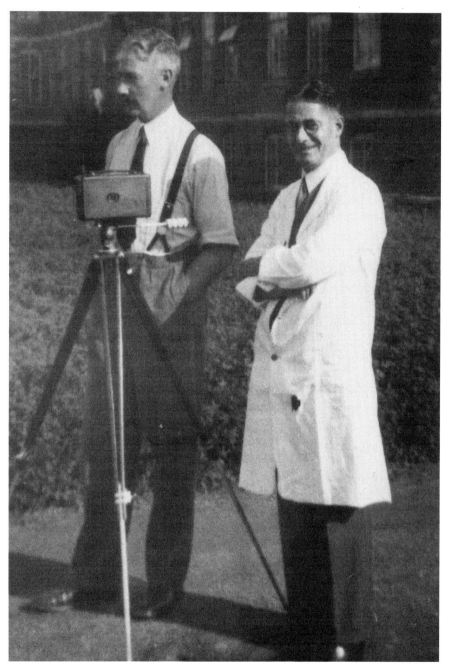

Figure 1. Howard Florey (right) *with A. Q. Wells filming excavations behind the Sir William Dunn School of Pathology in August 1939. Courtesy of the Sir William Dunn School of Pathology.*

Florey's long-standing interest in lysozyme, from his suggestion that Chain should study its mode of action, and from a survey by Chain of the literature on other antimicrobial products. Chain believed at that time that most of these substances were bacteriolytic enzymes, like lysozyme; and he undoubtedly became aware of the discovery by Dubos and Oswald Avery eight years earlier that an organism from the cranberry bogs of New Jersey produced an enzyme able to hydrolyze the capsular polysaccharide of the type III pneumococcus and to afford some protection to infected mice.

In the summer of 1939 war seemed imminent and members of the Sir William Dunn School of Pathology began excavations outside the laboratory to protect them from bombing. Florey was a keen photographer and he recorded this activity, accompanied by A. Q. Wells, who worked on tubercle and vole bacilli (fig. 1). Among the manual workers on this summer day were Norman Heatley, Robert Ebert (later a professor of medicine at Harvard), and Rolf Lium, an American clinician. The orders were given by B. G. Maegraith, an Australian member of the Territorial Army who subsequently became a professor of tropical medicine at Liverpool (fig. 2).

By this time, however, it had already been settled that Fleming's penicillin should be one of three microbial products to be studied. Apparently Florey was impressed by Fleming's demonstration of its activity against the staphylococcus (against which the sulfonamides were relatively ineffective) and Chain regarded its reported instability as a challenge to a biochemist. The war was certainly not responsible for this decision and the project was motivated by scientific interest and not by an expectation that the results would have clinical value. These are two points on which Florey and Chain were unreservedly agreed, although there were many later aspects of the penicillin story on which they took quite different views. Indeed, Chain wrote that his belief that penicillin was a protein led him to conclude that it could not be used systemically and Florey remarked later, "I don't think the idea of helping suffering humanity ever entered our minds."

Nevertheless, World War II greatly influenced the course of the Oxford penicillin project in a number of ways. The first was that Norman Heatley, who had intended to go to Denmark to study micromethods with Kaj Linderstrom-Lang, remained in the School of Pathology. After being asked by Florey to work on penicillin, with which Chain had made little progress, he devised a much more convenient assay than the one then in use. He suggested the transfer of penicillin from an organic solvent to an aqueous solution by a change of pH, a procedure which became an important step in purification. This provided material that was used later by Florey for his first experiments with mice in May 1940.

I mention these events because they seemed relevant to the title that Zanvil Cohn suggested, but I had no personal knowledge of most of them. In fact my first acquaintance with a therapeutic antibacterial substance was in September 1939 in Stockholm where I was a Rockefeller Foundation fellow in the laboratory of Hans von Euler. A Swedish physician gave me tablets of an early sulfonamide for a spreading streptococcal infection of the foot and told me that unless I took them I would only be going home, if at all, in a wooden box. But I managed to return alive to Oxford towards the end of the year and met Howard Florey for the first time, after being told by Sir Robert Robinson that he had an interesting proposal for research. Our interview was so brief that I received the impression that he had already decided to risk offering me a job.

The proposal was to work on wound shock. I did not sense any excitement about penicillin at that time, although Florey had already submitted applications to the Medical Research Council and the Rockefeller Foundation for financial support of a broad study of microbial antagonism by himself and Chain. In his description of the proposed biochemical aspects of the work, Chain had specifically mentioned penicillin together with an antibacterial product of *Pseudomonas* and the tyrothricin of Dubos. Despite the fact that the project had been conceived as an academic study, it is perhaps not surprising that attention was drawn to the possible therapeutic application of the substances concerned. In my experience those seeking financial support are rarely backward in suggesting that something of use may come from their research.

At this time I think that Howard Florey was waiting for further progress in the production of penicillin before undertaking experiments with laboratory animals. But two events may have persuaded him to bring these studies forward. In March 1940, J. M. Barnes, at Chain's request, tested the toxicity of a very crude preparation of penicillin in a mouse. About forty milligrams of this material (almost certainly less than 0.2% pure) produced no ill effect when given intraperitoneally. Florey may well have regarded this experiment as an encroachment on his own field and it did not demonstrate the remarkable lack of toxicity of pure penicillin. However, it did indicate that future biological studies with crude penicillin were unlikely to be complicated by major toxic impurities. A second event in March was Heatley's finding that penicillin with higher activity could be obtained by solvent transfer, although its purity was in fact still less than one percent.

Whatever the stimulus, Florey soon began studies which culminated in the mouse protection experiments between May and July. The result of the first experiment was so promising that he immediately decided to expand and intensify the work and asked me to collaborate with Chain in an attempt to isolate penicillin and determine its chemical nature.

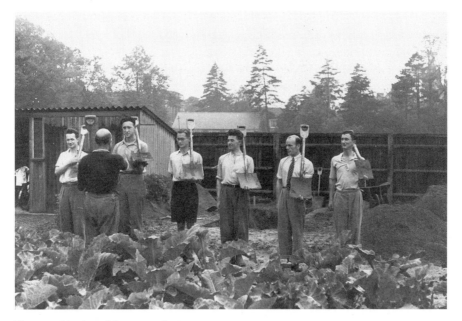

Figure 2.   Members of the Dunn School constructing bomb shelters. Robert Ebert (far left) *and Norman Heatley* (far right). *Courtesy of the Sir William Dunn School of Pathology.*

I will therefore now venture to say a little about our chemical and biochemical studies and how they impinged on the more biological ones and on Florey's activities. Despite his interest in the chemical nature of penicillin, Florey's overriding priority at that time was the production of enough for a small clinical trial. In the next chapter, Norman Heatley will describe how difficult it was in wartime Oxford to obtain enough material to treat even one or two patients. The problems were sometimes aggravated by contamination of the cultures of *Penicillium notatum* with bacteria producing a penicillinase. This enzyme had been discovered in *Escherichia coli* by Chain and me in 1940, while we were looking for an enzyme that might account for the poor activity of penicillin against gram-negative bacteria, but too little penicillin was then available for us to throw light on its mode of action.

One attempt by Chain to deal with contamination when Florey and Heatley were later in America is amusing in retrospect. He ordered the departmental workshop to make large numbers of metal caps for the vessels then used for surface culture of the *Penicillium*. They undoubtedly excluded bacteria, but they also impeded the entry of oxygen and no penicillin was produced. On another occasion, I remember, a lead-containing metal tube was introduced into makeshift equipment for handling active culture fluids. None of the penicillin that entered the tube was ever found again. Later we showed that a number of heavy metal ions, including lead and copper, catalyzed a rapid inactivation of the antibiotic. A different type of disconcerting event occurred in January 1941 when the first patient ever to receive crude penicillin intravenously later developed a sharp rise in temperature and a rigor, and a second patient reacted similarly. But this problem was quickly overcome by chromatographic purification.

Soon after the gratifying results of the first clinical trial, Heatley went with Florey to the United States and Canada and worked first at the Northern Regional Research Laboratory, U.S. Department of Agriculture, in Peoria and then at Merck. Florey made unceasing attempts, both in the U.K. and the U.S., to obtain larger amounts of penicillin for further trials. What was the outcome of these endeavors? Research in the United States at Peoria and in pharmaceutical companies revolutionized the production of penicillin by the introduction of deep fermentation, new culture media, and new strains of *Penicillium*. The fact that the project was supported by substantial amounts of money from the American government was attributed partly by Florey to his friendship with A. N. Richards, who had become chairman of the Committee on Medical Research of the Office of Scientific Research and Development, and who respected Florey's judgment.

Nevertheless, despite Florey's hopes, very little American penicillin came to him. About six years later, when I was returning from my first visit to the United States and went to Merck, I was astonished to be told that George Merck himself wanted to see me. It turned out that he wished me to assure Florey that Merck's failure to fulfill its undertaking to supply him with penicillin was not due to any lack of good will, but to the fact that supplies were commandeered by the army after the entry of America into the war in December 1941. However, with material from British sources, including the Dunn School in which an extraction plant was put together by A. G. Sanders from equipment used in the dairy industry, Howard and Ethel Florey were able to carry out a highly successful second clinical trial.

In early 1943 Florey and Hugh Cairns, an Australian neurosurgeon who had worked with Harvey Cushing as a Rockefeller fellow and had become an Oxford professor and a brigadier in the Army Medical Service, went to North Africa to help determine how very small amounts of crude penicillin could be used to the best advantage in the treatment of war wounds. The bold step was taken to suture early severe soft tissue wounds infected with gram-positive bacteria and to introduce penicillin through tubes stitched into stab holes (fig. 3). This procedure appears to have reduced the development of dangerous sepsis and to have greatly promoted healing.

Towards the end of the year Florey went to Moscow with Sanders on a joint Anglo-American medical mission. He advised that the best way for the Russians

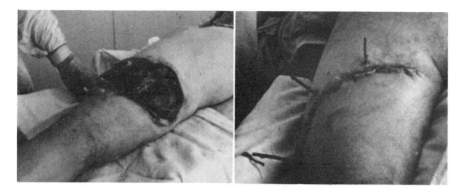

Figure 3. (Left) *A war wound in the North African campaign.* (Right) *Local treatment by early suture and instillation of penicillin. From a motion picture taken by Howard Florey in 1943. Courtesy of the Sir William Dunn School of Pathology.*

to learn how to produce penicillin was for them to visit plants in Britain and the U.S. Not surprisingly there proved to be serious impediments to the implementation of this suggestion. Its earliest outcome appeared two years later, when a Soviet biologist arrived in the Dunn School. For some months he made a colorful addition to the department and he undoubtedly enjoyed his stay, but he learned little about how to set up a penicillin plant.

When Florey visited pharmaceutical companies in the U.S. and Canada in 1941, he found that Merck, Squibb, and Pfizer proposed to become seriously involved in the penicillin project but that a number of firms "showed little interest and some none at all." One reason for a lack of unanimous enthusiasm was undoubtedly the formidable difficulty, at that time, of producing penicillin by fermentation. But another may well have been the expectation that penicillin would be produced more easily by chemical synthesis. For this to be possible, of course, its structure had first to be determined.

From the beginning Florey was eager for Chain and me to pursue our chemical studies. By the end of 1941 we had obtained a penicillin preparation which was about fifty percent pure and Florey was happy to find that it was even less toxic, though far more active, than the material used in the first clinical trial. In the following year we began to collaborate with Robinson, one of the great organic chemists of his day, and Wilson Baker in the Dyson Perrins laboratory (fig. 4), and later with John Cornforth and others. In the Dunn School we isolated characteristic degradation products of penicillin, although an erroneous microanalyst's report delayed our finding of sulfur in the molecule until July 1943. I have a vivid memory of Florey asking from time to time, "Any crystals today?" and

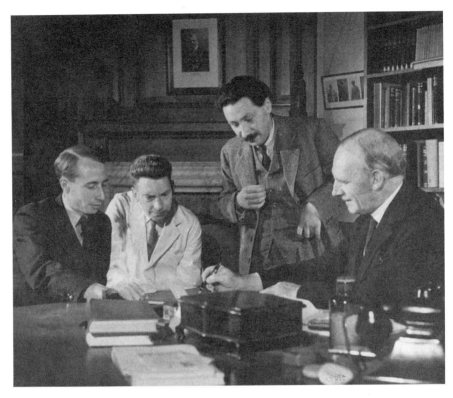

Figure 4. Chemical collaborators at Oxford. (Left to right) *Edward Abraham, Wilson Baker, Ernst Chain, and Robert Robinson. Courtesy of the Sir William Dunn School of Pathology.*

having to reply, "Not yet." But in August the Medical Research Council in London was informed that a crystalline sodium salt of penicillin had been obtained by Harold MacPhillamy, Oskar Wintersteiner, and Joseph Alicino at Squibb. Our own purest material at that time had been isolated for chemical work as a nonhygroscopic barium salt, but on receipt of the exciting American news I converted it to a sodium salt and this formed a syrup that crystallized spontaneously. It then became clear that the Oxford and American penicillins, produced in different media, had different side chains. They were named F and G, respectively, although a nomenclature beginning with F was not pleasing to Chain for reasons that you may be able to guess.

By October 1943 our knowledge of the degradation products and particularly the physicochemical properties of penicillin convinced me that it had a β-lactam structure and I proposed this structure to Chain (fig. 5, *top*). However,

Robinson felt certain that penicillin had a thiazolidine-oxazolone structure (fig. 5, *bottom*) which differed in the way in which ring closure had occurred. He was not a man who would readily accept ideas that conflicted with his own and this led to a controversy that ended only when Dorothy Crowfoot Hodgkin and Barbara Low revealed the β-lactam structure by x-ray crystallography.

By 1943 the study of the chemistry of penicillin had developed into a remarkable and confidential Anglo-American project in which similar findings were made independently on both sides of the Atlantic. Nevertheless, despite the combined efforts of about forty major academic and commercial organizations, only a trace of synthetic penicillin had been obtained by the end of the war and that by a process designed to synthesize the wrong structure. A few years later John Sheehan accomplished a notable rational synthesis of penicillin at MIT, after introducing a new reagent to close the β-lactam ring. By then the astonishing increase in the yields obtained from strains of *Penicillium chrysogenum* had made it unlikely that total synthesis would ever compete commercially with fermentation. But chemical studies bore fruit later, when clinically valuable semisynthetic penicillins and cephalosporins began to be produced from the penicillin nucleus and the cephalosporin nucleus, respectively.

Before ending this digression I should like to mention that the Rockefeller laboratories had not been entirely detached from the penicillin project. In 1945 they contributed a description of a spectroscopic assay to the twelve hundred or more confidential reports on the chemistry of penicillin that were circulated during the war. They saw the birth of Lyman Craig's method of countercurrent distribution between solvents for the purification of natural products and this enabled Vincent du Vigneaud and his group to obtain crystalline penicillin from trivial amounts of a synthetic product. And it now seems likely that a tripeptide from which both penicillins and cephalosporins are derived is synthesized, like gramicidin, by a nonribosomal multienzyme mechanism analogous to that revealed here more than thirty years ago by Fritz Lipmann and elaborated by Horst Kleinkauf, Hans von Dohren, and others.

By the end of the war it seemed that the value and limitations of penicillin had been clearly defined, but in the early 1950s there were indications that its great contribution to chemotherapy would decline because penicillinase-producing staphylococci were becoming prevalent in hospitals. Two unforeseen events, however, were to change the outlook at that time. One was the isolation of the penicillin nucleus (6-APA) and the other the discovery of cephalosporin C and the preparation of its nucleus (7-ACA).

Convincing evidence for the existence of the penicillin nucleus in fermentation fluids was first obtained in Japan by K. Sakaguchi and S. Murao in 1950 and

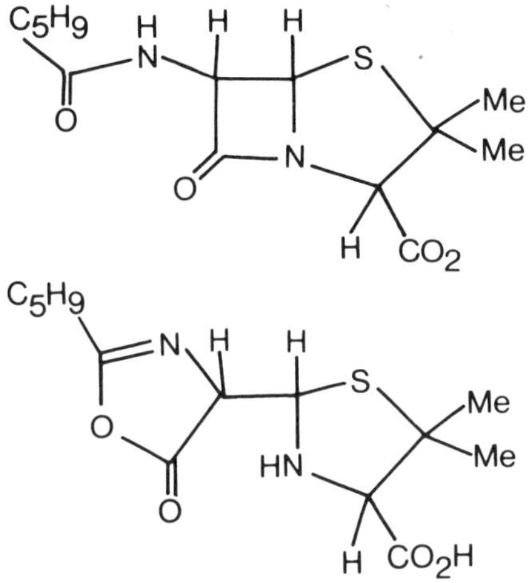

Figure 5. The β-lactam structure (top) *and thiazolidine-oxazolone structure* (bottom) *proposed for penicillin F.*

by T. Kato in 1953. They did not pursue their findings, but in 1958 G. Rolinson and R. Batchelor from the Beecham Company independently made observations similar to those of Kato while working in Chain's laboratory in Rome. After their return to Beecham, 6-APA was isolated and a series of new semisynthetic penicillins was prepared by coupling it chemically with different side chains. One of the first of these, methicillin, was active against staphylococci that were resistant to the earlier penicillins.

My colleague Guy Newton and I discovered cephalosporin C in 1953 among the products of a strain of *Cephalosporium ácremonium* that had been isolated from the sea in 1945 by Giuseppe Brotzu near a sewage outfall at Cagliari, Sardinia. Brotzu, a professor of hygiene and a politician, published the results of his work locally in a paper entitled "Ricerche su di un nuovo antibiotico" and believed that his crude extract was useful for the treatment of typhoid fever. He tried to interest an Italian pharmaceutical company, but without success, and in 1948 sent a culture of the *Cephalosporium* to Oxford. It turned out eventually that this organism produced not one but at least five different antibiotics. My main attention focused on a labile water-soluble substance with a broad range of activity, not because I imagined that it would be clinically useful but because it seemed to belong to a group of relatively unstable peptides in which I had long been interested from an academic point of view. Newton and I showed that it was a new type of penicillin with an amino acid side chain and it was named penicillin N (fig. 6, *top*). This penicillin was undoubtedly mainly responsible for the activity described by Brotzu.

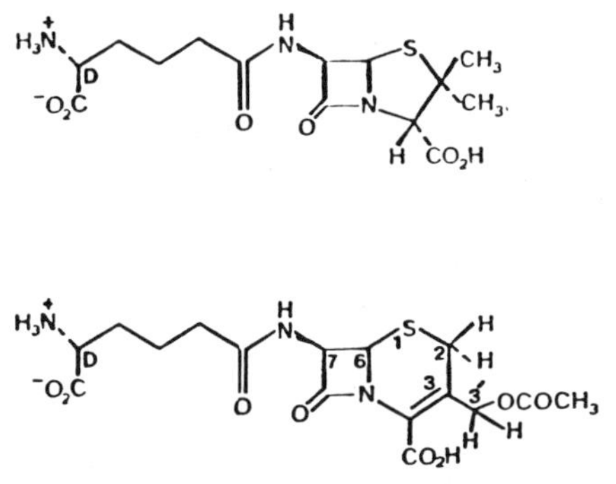

Figure 6. Structure of penicillin N (top) and cephalosporin C (bottom).

During our chemical studies of penicillin N we came to realize that purified preparations were still contaminated with a small amount of another substance. The latter was finally isolated as a crystalline sodium salt and named cephalosporin C. Only then was it shown to have antibacterial activity. This substance—the first of the cephalosporins as they are now known—aroused our interest, not only because it resembled penicillin N in some chemical respects but not in others, but because it was resistant to a staphylococcal penicillinase. After prolonged chemical study I was convinced by 1958 that its structure was that shown in figure 6 (*bottom*). Not everyone at first believed this structure, but it was soon confirmed by an x-ray crystallographic analysis by Dorothy Hodgkin and E. Maslen.

Florey showed that cephalosporin C was even less toxic than penicillin G to mice and that it could protect mice from infections with penicillin-resistant staphylococci. We obtained small amounts of the nucleus of this molecule (7-ACA) by treating cephalosporin C with dilute acid and found, as expected, that more active compounds could be obtained by coupling new side chains with this nucleus. However, the yields of 7-ACA obtained were too low for our process to be commercially feasible. This problem was later solved in the Lilly Research Laboratories and the door was thus opened for the semisynthesis of many thousands of cephalosporins for biological study.

Let me now conclude with some general remarks on Howard Florey and his role in the penicillin saga. Florey was a physiologist and a highly skilled experimenter with laboratory animals. He would probably have studied chemistry instead of medicine had there not been a poor outlook for jobs in chemistry in Australia when he was young. But he retained a particular interest in the nature of chemical substances with biological activity and set out to give pathology "a good twist away from diagnosis and morbid anatomy." He had no high opinion of clinical research at that time and it was his belief that pathology would benefit by joining with other disciplines which set the stage in Oxford for the discovery of the clinical value of penicillin. His view that a study of antimicrobial products from natural sources would be of scientific interest has survived the test of time.

Florey was reserved and sometimes quick-tempered in his most vigorous years. His limited skill in diplomacy before he mellowed in later life may have contributed to the deplorable quality of much of the publicity which followed the demonstration of the therapeutic power of penicillin. But two characteristics led to my growing liking for him and I shall always remember them with gratitude. He was essentially a modest man, who never forgot the good fortune that had attended the decision to work on penicillin, and to whom one could easily voice an opinion that differed from his own. And he never failed to draw attention to the role of his junior colleagues or to show concern for their welfare. In his handling of the penicillin problem he showed a great ability to organize research, although he once said to me that the Dunn School was filled with prima donnas. Whether he made this remark at a time when he was not seeing eye-to-eye with Chain, I can no longer remember. But it is clear that he did all he could to further Chain's career during the latter's early years in Oxford.

PENICILLIN AND LUCK

Norman G. Heatley

Sixty years ago, when I was a student at Cambridge, England, I most days passed a building at the corner of Downing and Corn Exchange Streets on the walls of which was incised in large capitals Louis Pasteur's stern warning LE HASARD NE FAVORISE QUE CEUX QUI SONT PREPARES (Luck only favors those who are prepared). I took this to heart, and later was equally impressed by Paul Ehrlich's opinion that successful research required the four Gs: *geschick* (skill), *geduld* (patience), *geld* (money), and *glück* (luck). Unfortunately he did not explain how to acquire the last of these. It seems to me that luck—and I mean good luck, or serendipity—has played an interesting part in the early history of penicillin, and I would like to offer some examples.

But first I must declare and acknowledge my own enormous luck in finding myself in Howard Florey's laboratory at the Sir William Dunn School of Pathology, Oxford, in 1936; and from 1939 having the privilege of working personally with him and his colleagues on penicillin. Strangely, that was not my first contact with penicillin because in 1934 or 1935, while in F. Gowland Hopkins's Biochemical Laboratory, Cambridge, I attended a Tea Club lecture on selective enzyme inhibitors. In the discussion afterwards the lecturer was asked if any other selec-

Emeritus, Sir William Dunn School of Pathology, University of Oxford. Worked with Howard Florey on the isolation, production, and standardization of penicillin.

tive inhibitors were known; the answer included ". . . and penicillin, a curious fungal product described by A. Fleming." My curiosity was aroused and I took some trouble to consult what is now Fleming's famous 1929 paper in *The British Journal of Experimental Pathology* (1) and to make notes on it. So when Florey spoke to me for the first time about penicillin in 1939 I at least knew what he was talking about.

To start at the beginning, here is a photograph (fig. 1) of Fleming's famous plate, the essentials being a staphylococcal plate culture contaminated by a fungus from which something is diffusing which is clearly affecting the bacterial colonies; this something turned out to be penicillin. Most would agree that Fleming was very lucky to have this demonstration, set up and completed by Nature herself, displayed before him; but I would maintain that it was also fortunate that it was disclosed to *him*, since he was particularly well-equipped to detect and interpret its significance. An adept experimenter, usually with the simplest apparatus such as the slide cell, the teat and capillary tube, and the artificial wound, he was also interested in the more bizarre aspects of bacteriology—witness his "paintings" on nutrient media inoculated with pigmented bacteria that developed on incubation. No doubt his acute powers of observation must have been reinforced by his previous discovery of lysozyme. Let us consider the actual scenario of his discovery of penicillin, with regard to the research of the late Ronald Hare, as described in his book *The Birth of Penicillin and the Disarming of Microbes* (2).

In the summer of 1928 Fleming goes on holiday, unaware that he has been chosen by the Fates to take the first steps in introducing the antibiotics to mankind. Having made a wise choice of their agent, the Fates also arranged that one of his plates, inoculated with staphylococci but not incubated, should be contaminated with a spore of *Penicillium notatum*, and that the weather during subsequent weeks should provide the sequence of rather narrow temperature ranges required to produce the penicillin effect. Fleming returns from his holiday and goes through the pile of used plates on his bench, looking at them and discarding them into the tray of disinfectant. The plates are many, and soon they are piled up, clear of the disinfectant. But what is this? Gracious Heavens, he has discarded *the* plate! All is not lost, for the Fates have a messenger on hand in the form of Fleming's colleague, D. M. Pryce. Pryce makes his entrance, they chat about staphylococci and, to make a point, Fleming picks up some of the discarded plates. The Fates hold their breath. Yes! He picks up *the* plate, looks at it, and says "That's funny . . ." How fortunate that trays rather than buckets were used for discarded cultures and that D. M. Pryce was on hand at the critical moment.

Now for a little wild speculation. Before Hare's work mentioned above, which was published in 1970, it was sometimes said that had Fleming not

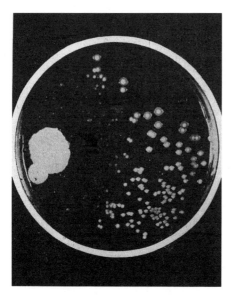

Figure 1. Fleming's famous plate, showing staphylococcal colonies affected by something (penicillin) diffusing from the contaminating fungus. Originally published in The British Journal of Experimental Pathology, *1929, 10:226.*

made his discovery, someone else would soon have done so "because the time was ripe." But taking Hare's work into consideration, the chances of another spontaneous display of the effect seen by Fleming would seem to be very low. The phenomenon is simple, and surely anyone with the most limited microbial expertise should have been able to recognize and interpret it (though against this assertion it must be said that even Fleming himself missed it the first time around). The effect could theoretically have been generated at any time after 1881, when Robert Koch introduced media solidified with agar. But the fact remains that it was nearly fifty years after that date that Fleming made his discovery, although many other examples of microbial antagonism had been described during that time. And now another sixty years have passed. Has the effect ever been reported again? Or perhaps observed, but not reported? Or dare one speculate that the chances of another spontaneous occurrence of the phenomenon are so slight that so far it may have been a "one-off" occurrence. And this in spite of the probability that since the early 1940s *Penicillium notatum* has become a much more common component of at least some laboratory environments.

Compared with the heroic displays of luck at the end of the 1920s, its contribution ten years later to the work at Oxford was very low key, and to some extent related to the fact that Britain was at war. Because of this, the availability of laboratory and other equipment was capricious. For example, at one period the ordinary empty soft drink bottle became a prized possession, since a bottle of squash, if one were lucky enough to find one in a shop, would only be sold in exchange for an empty one. Thus the fortuitous acquisition of a large number of identical strong glass bottles early in the war aroused curiosity and mild satisfaction at the time but later was seen to have been a stroke of major good fortune. They had a capacity of 4.5 liters, were stable, could be picked up and held by one

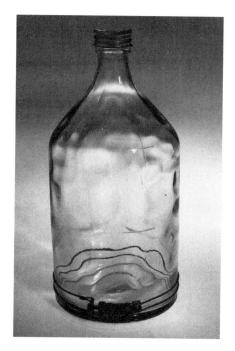

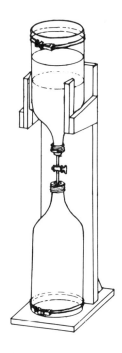

Figure 2.   A good supply of these strong glass bottles of unknown origin proved valuable for the laboratory large-scale working up of penicillin. Note oc-
cludable air hole near base.

Figure 3.   An inverted bottle held in a wooden
stand being used as a separating funnel.

Buchner funnel

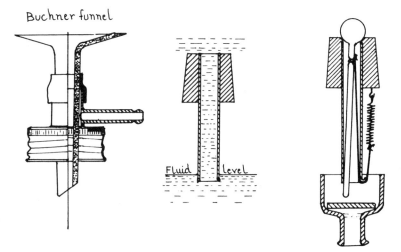

Fluid   level

Figure 4.   (Left) Metal cap of a bottle modified for suction filtration. (Center) Constant level automatic
filtration from an inverted bottle not shown in diagram. (Right) Arrangement for preventing escape of
fluid from an inverted bottle.

hand, and could be adapted for a number of purposes (fig. 2). Solvent transfer became a key process in the extraction and purification of penicillin, but large separating funnels were virtually unobtainable; with a minor adaptation a bottle provided a rugged and more convenient substitute:

⇥⋘- A small hole was drilled near the bottom. (A minor piece of luck was that one of Florey's team was interested in the art of china riveting and had the necessary equipment for drilling holes in glass.) The hole was normally closed by a cork pad controlled by a screw passing through a brass block held in place by a wire harness. The two immiscible phases (perhaps acidified crude penicillin and amyl acetate) were placed in the bottle and shaken. The plain cork bung was then replaced by one carrying a glass tube with a tap (or a tap substitute) and the bottle was inverted in a simple wooden stand (fig. 3). The cork pad was released, allowing air to enter, and when the phases had settled the lower layer was run off into another bottle in the usual way; if this also had the air-hole modification, a washing or back extraction could be carried out in the same bottle.

⇥⋘- For automatic filtration the bottle of filtrand was fitted with a bung carrying a short wide glass tube (fig. 4, *center*). When the bottle was inverted over the filter funnel, liquid escaped in spurts interspersed with gulps of air entering the bottle, until the level of fluid in the funnel just reached the end of the tube. This simple, well-known, constant level arrangement allowed the filtration to be completed without attention, and as the two bottles were the same size there was no risk of overflowing.

⇥⋘- Suction could be applied, as for a Buchner funnel, through a modified screw cap (fig. 4, *left*) for the lower, receiving bottle.

⇥⋘- The bottles were also used as reservoirs in a rather complicated countercurrent extraction apparatus, the same constant level system providing a steady delivery pressure (fig. 4, *right*). Complete avoidance of spillage when a bottle was inverted—important if the bottle contained ten percent phosphoric acid—was achieved by a ball on the end of a glass rod being held by a stainless steel spring against the rim of the hole in the base of the bung. Only as the bottle was lowered the last centimeter or so on its stand was the ball pushed up by the rod, allowing fluid to emerge.

Cultivation of the fungus was simple. Medium, to a depth of 1–2 centimeters, was sterilized in a container closed by a cotton plug. With full aseptic precautions it was inoculated with spores of *Penicillium notatum* and incubated at 24–26°C for about ten days. The medium, which by then had become bright yellow and contained penicillin, was harvested from under the fungal mat. Because of the long incubation period it followed that if the target was to set up and harvest, say, thirty vessels per day, then at least three hundred vessels would be required. All kinds of containers were pressed into service—flasks, bottles, trays,

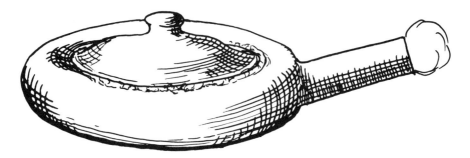

Figure 5. Sixteen of these old-fashioned bedpans, borrowed from the Radcliffe Infirmary, were among the assorted vessels used for early cultivation of the fungus.

pie dishes, tins, and hospital bedpans (fig. 5). There may be a resonance here since the bedpans can be likened to enormous Carrel flasks, a utensil invented, I believe, in The Rockefeller Institute; they must have been very common during this period.

These assorted culture vessels were very uneconomical of incubator and autoclave space and of labor, but by the end of May 1940 enough penicillin was available for Florey to set up a mouse protection experiment. It was a good example of the kind of simple, well-planned experiment giving clear-cut results which appealed to Florey (fig. 6), and I would like to summarize it as follows: eight mice were each given an intraperitoneal injection of virulent streptococci. One hour later, two were given, subcutaneously, a single dose of ten milligrams of a certain penicillin preparation. Two others were given five milligrams then and four further doses, each of five milligrams, at 3, 5, 7, and 11 hours after infection. The other four mice, the controls, received no penicillin. About 7 hours later the controls looked very sick and died between 13 and 17 hours after infection. All the treated mice looked relatively well. Those receiving the single dose survived for four and six days, while of those receiving the larger, divided dose one died after six days and the other remained well until killed some weeks later.

This was most encouraging and the next day, a Sunday, future plans were discussed. The mouse protection experiment would have to be repeated and extended with different pathogenic bacteria, and the chemistry, pharmacology, and antibacterial properties pursued ever more vigorously. But the greatest need was to try to step up production since the yield was pathetically low: 1–2 units per milliliter of culture fluid or, in terms of pure penicillin, not more than one milligram per liter. Even at this time Florey was aware that penicillin would have to be tested in human patients before its manufacture could be seriously considered, but as he pointed out, a man is three thousand times as big as a mouse.

In peacetime this would be the stage at which one would seek a commercial firm to grow the fungus on a pilot plant scale, but in wartime firms had full order books and it was understandable that they should have been reluctant to devote scarce resources to the possibly difficult production of a material which was only potentially valuable. The answer was to try to grow sufficient penicillin at the Dunn School, and one of the most urgent needs was for a supply of better culture vessels. A large chemical glassware manufacturing firm was approached. Yes, they could make the glass vessels to our specification, but the mold alone would cost about five hundred pounds and delivery time would be about six months. This was a blow; at best six months seemed a very long time, and delivery could easily have dragged on indefinitely. Someone then had the idea of a ceramic vessel, perhaps made by the slipcast process. In this process the object to be copied, a teapot, say,

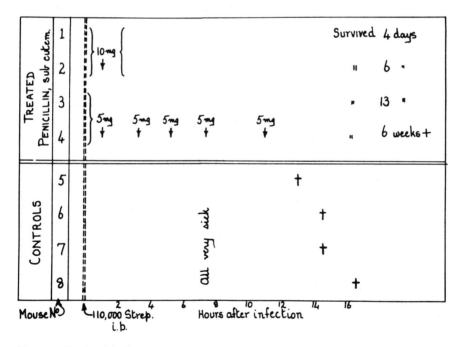

Figure 6. Results of the first mouse protection experiment set up by Florey on Saturday, May 25, 1940.

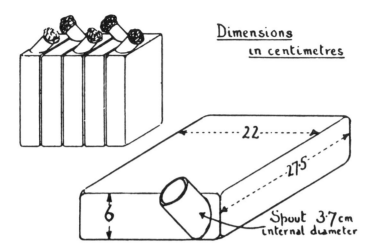

Figure 7. The ceramic culture vessels specially made by James Macintyre & Co. Ltd., Burslem.

is embedded in a porous mold which can be taken apart and reassembled after removing the pattern—in this case the teapot. The cavity is then filled with a thick suspension of clay, known as slip. The porous mold sucks out water from the slip which is in contact with it and after a suitable time the liquid slip is poured out, leaving a layer of semisolid slip lining the cavity in the form of the original teapot. After this has become firmer it is removed from the mold, dried, and fired. The process is relatively cheap, whether for many or a few copies.

The piece of luck I have been leading up to is that when the idea of a ceramic vessel was brought up Florey said, with excitement, that he knew a physician in The Potteries, J. P. Stock, to whom he would write immediately. Stock replied by telegram that the only firm likely to be able to help was James Macintyre & Co. Ltd. of Burslem. The next day I was sent to Burslem and was amazed to find that during the three or four days that they had had our sketches they had actually made—not fired, of course—three prototypes, one of which was almost exactly what was needed. Minor corrections were made with the help of a pocket knife and three sample vessels were promised eighteen days later, the apparent delay being due to the several days required for firing in the tunnel kiln. The sample vessels arrived punctually on time and a trial run showed that penicillin was produced satisfactorily in them. A firm order was placed and the first batch of 174 vessels was fetched on 23 December 1940. Half of them were washed and sterilized the next day, and on Christmas Day were seeded with spores of the fungus, about two months after first contacting Macintyre & Co. The number of days of *avoidable* delay during that period must have been very few, perhaps nil. Each vessel held one liter of medium in a layer 1.7 centimeters deep, and they could be stacked vertically for autoclaving and inoculation, and horizontally for incubation (figs. 7 and 8); over seven hundred were made eventually. Without Florey's acquaintance with Stock, and Stock's introduction to Macintyre & Co., the search for a firm willing to make the ceramic vessels would almost certainly have been fruitless.

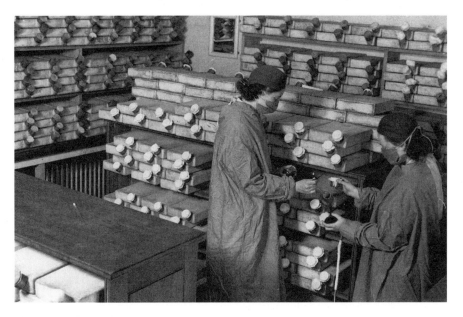

Figure 8. Cultures of Penicillium notatum *stacked in the operating theater of the Sir William Dunn School of Pathology, Oxford, which could be held at 24°C, a satisfactory temperature for the production of penicillin.*

There had never been any indication that penicillin was toxic to mice, but when a human volunteer received one hundred milligrams of a preparation of which ten milligrams had had no visible effect on a mouse, she sustained a rigor. The same happened with a different volunteer. Was the rigor due to one or more impurities, or was it due to the active principle? If the latter, its clinical value would have been partially or wholly vitiated. The question was quickly answered by Edward Abraham, who showed that chromatography on alumina would separate the pyrogen(s) from the penicillin, as well as providing a purer and more active preparation. By good luck penicillin itself is not pyrogenic.

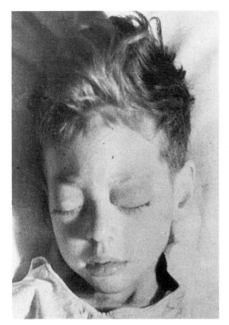 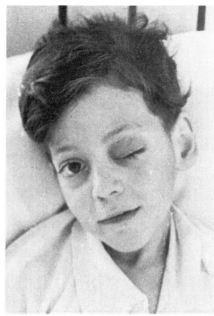

Figure 9. (Left) *Case No. 4, one of the first six gravely ill patients to be treated parenterally with penicillin, just before start of penicillin treatment.* (Right) Eleven days after start of penicillin treatment (The Lancet, *August 16, 1941*).

With the new ceramic culture vessels coming on stream, penicillin became a little more freely available, and within a year of the first mouse protection experiment six gravely ill patients had been treated with penicillin at the Radcliffe Infirmary, Oxford, with Charles Fletcher of the Infirmary acting as liaison officer with the Dunn School. The response was striking, so I will briefly mention just one of these six cases. The patient was a four-and-a-half-year old boy diagnosed as suffering from a staphylococcal-induced cavernous sinus thrombosis, a condition almost invariably fatal. He had not responded to sulfapyridine and just before the beginning of penicillin treatment (fig. 9, *left*) he appeared moribund. After nine days of treatment he had almost recovered; figure 9 (*right*) was taken eleven days after beginning of treatment. Unhappily he died from a ruptured mycotic aneurism, but an autopsy was permitted which confirmed the diagnosis and showed that the lesion was resolving, with the generation of healthy granulation tissue. Gordon Stewart in his book *The Penicillin Group of Drugs* (3) comments on these six cases with admirable conciseness:

The results were convincing, each in a different way, and the absence of toxicity was almost as impressive as the rapid therapeutic effect. . . . In the present day, when a clinical trial is becoming an exercise in statistics and bureaucracy, there is irony in the reflection that the massive efforts which followed were based upon a few toxicity tests in rodents, and upon a clinical trial in six selected subjects, two of whom died. Had the toxicity tests been extended to guinea pigs, penicillin might have been rejected; had current regulations been in force, it would have been ineligible for submission.

I think Stewart is referring here to the British Committee on the Safety of Medicines, a much-respected body of distinguished experts which was established in the 1960s. Is it too whimsical to suggest that our greatest piece of luck might be the fact that this worthy body did not exist in 1941?

References

1. Fleming, A. 1929. On the antibacterial action of cultures of a Penicillium, with special reference to their use in the isolation of *B. influenzae. British Journal of Experimental Pathology.* 10:226.
2. Hare, R. 1970. *The Birth of Penicillin and the Disarming of Microbes.* London: George Allen & Unwin Ltd.
3. Stewart, G. T. 1965. *The Penicillin Group of Drugs.* London: Elsevier Science Publishing Co. Inc.

CHLORAMPHENICOL, KUALA LUMPUR, AND THE FIRST THERAPEUTIC CONQUESTS OF SCRUB TYPHUS AND TYPHOID FEVER

Theodore E. Woodward

Unfortunately, the late Joe Smadel cannot relate the story of the Scrub Typhus Mission to Kuala Lumpur, Malaya, in 1948. He was the architect of these trials to test the efficacy of chloromycetin, the first broad-spectrum antibiotic. Freshly commissioned as a Captain, Joe was assigned to the Walter Reed Army Institute for Research (WRAIR) in September 1941, coming from The Rockefeller Institute for Medical Research. After a brief meeting there, our friendship was cemented in Naples, Italy, when he, along with Yale Kneeland and Emory Cushing, came from the London headquarters of the European Theatre of Operations (ETO) to observe the measures applied to control the typhus epidemic. We exchanged information regarding efficacy of killed typhus vaccines and that only one or two doses were protective. Also, we discussed the importance of antibody response as a crude index of protection. Later, I was scolded by my commanding officer in Italy for allowing such important scientific information escape to another command. The mission of this team of officers was to observe and advise the Chief Surgeon of ETO regarding control of louse-borne typhus fever in order to cope with the anticipated epidemic threat after Germany's capitulation.

After the armistice, Joe became scientific director of WRAIR and functioned as a pillar of scientific support for various commissions of the Armed

Professor Emeritus, University of Maryland. Discovered, with Joseph Smadel during clinical trials in the Far East, that chloramphenicol cures typhus and typhoid fever.

Forces Epidemiological Board, including Rickettsial Diseases, Immunization, Virus Diseases, Epidemic Hemorrhagic Fever, and Epidemiological Survey.

During this post-WWII period, P. R. Burkholder, of Yale, noted in 1947 that the growth of adjacent inocula of both gram-positive and -negative bacteria was inhibited on agar streak cultures by a new actinomycete isolated from the soil of a mulched field near Caracas, Venezuela. From culture filtrates of this new soil organism, later named *Streptomyces venezuelae,* a crystalline antibiotic was isolated that was inhibitory for a wide range of gram-positive and -negative bacteria, rickettsiae, and the psittacosis virus. Its unusually broad range of antimicrobial action, low toxicity for animals, great stability, and effective absorption from the gastrointestinal tract suggested that chloramphenicol, as it was called, might become the first major antibiotic for clinical use since the discovery of streptomycin.

Indeed, this prediction was borne out by the early clinical trials, soon to be discussed, which were carried out in Kuala Lumpur, Malaya. These pioneering studies established chloramphenicol as the first drug of real value for treatment of rickettsial infections and typhoid fever. Its usefulness for treatment of numerous bacterial infections was rapidly recognized, and in this manner, chloramphenicol was ushered in as the first member of the series of so-called broad-spectrum antibiotics.

The unique composition of chloramphenicol (i.e., the presence of organically bound chlorine and a nitro group, which are uncommonly found in naturally occurring compounds) was recognized early by the Parke, Davis & Co. chemists. This group later elucidated the structure of the antibiotic and developed a method for the synthesis that was suitable for commercial production.

Chloramphenicol was shown to be rapidly absorbed from the gastrointestinal tract, to attain therapeutic concentration in the blood quickly, and to diffuse readily into the cerebral spinal fluid and other body fluids. The antibiotic appeared to be conjugated and degraded, mostly in the liver, and largely excreted in both active and inactive forms in the urine and in the bile and saliva in therapeutic amounts. Chloramphenicol appeared to penetrate some body cells in a form with antimicrobial activity.

To return to the scenario: scrub typhus fever remained an enigma, there was no vaccine, and therapy with paraaminobenzoic acid was awkward. Joe relentlessly pursued leads for better specific therapy. On Joe's prior request, Fred Stimpert of Parke, Davis & Co. provided him samples of any antimicrobial agent showing inhibitory properties for rickettsiae. Chloromycetin was included in a batch of possible candidates. With Betsy Jackson, this new streptomyces-derived

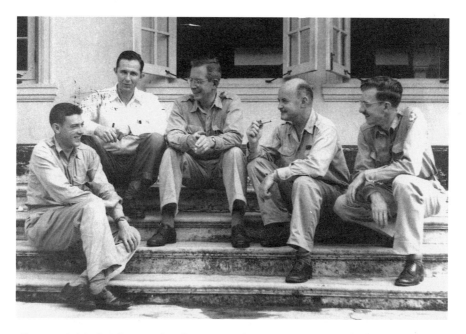

Figure 1. Original Malayan scrub typhus team. (Left to right) *Robert Traub, Theodore E. Woodward, Director Joseph E. Smadel, Cornelius Philip, and Herb L. Ley, Jr.*

antibiotic was shown to inhibit *Rickettsia orientalis* (scrub typhus) and lymphopathia venereum infection in fertile hens' eggs and mice. Joe and Herb Ley successfully treated a few cases of typhus in Mexico and demonstrated that blood levels of chloromycetin occurred after oral administration.

During this period, I migrated from Baltimore to WRAIR each Thursday to escape the rigors of clinical practice and exchange ideas about treatment of rickettsial diseases, including the use of PABA.

Through authorities at WRAIR and the respective Ministries and Department of State, Joe arranged the mission to Kuala Lumpur for testing the efficacy of chloromycetin in scrub typhus. Raymond Lewthwaite, director of the Institute for Medical Research, Kuala Lumpur, graciously approved the proposal. Later, this remarkable man, himself an authority in the field of rickettsial diseases, became a colleague and close friend of the team. Joe selected the group shown in figure 1: Herb Ley, scientific laboratory assistant to Joe; Cornelius (Neil) Philip and Robert (Bob) Traub, entomologists; and myself as clinician. The contract, funded by the Medical Research and Development Command through the Commission on Immunization, was awarded to the University of Maryland School of

Medicine. On one occasion, Stanhope Bayne-Jones quipped that this contract "was conceived in inequity and executed in sin" and retorted promptly that "it got things done."

A special military transport plane carried the team and essential equipment. Several spicy incidents relieved the monotony of the long journey across the Pacific to Singapore. Joe held a royal straight flush in diamonds in the Hamilton Air Force Terminal. We immediately froze the deck. Later, in Kwajelein, a near-rupture of the small unit almost occurred. The island

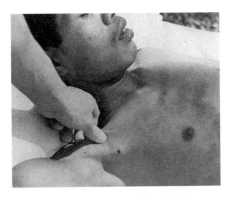

Figure 2. First patient treated with chloromycetin showing primary lesion (eschar) in axilla with local adenopathy.

was a highly restricted area because of pending nuclear testing. One of the team members, in spite of careful instructions, failed to make the passenger count at time of departure. The Air Force pilot, a lieutenant colonel, was irate and Joe was livid. Temperature inside the cabin exceeded 110 degrees. It was increased by 30 degrees with Joe's crisp verbiage when our wandering scientist returned with a new species of grasshopper taken from a red restricted area across the landing strip.

Lewthwaite met the plane in Singapore on Sunday, March 14, 1948. The Sunday holiday precluded removal of the jeeps and other heavy equipment by airport personnel. Steaming and undaunted, Joe was bursting for action and practically built a makeshift block and tackle for the purpose. We immediately motored through the green Malayan rain forest with its rubber plantations and isolated tin mines to the Selangor capital of Kuala Lumpur.

Unbelievably, before a change of clothes, Lewthwaite took us to the bedside of a young Malayan soldier named Mohammed Osman who had acquired his illness near the air strip in Kuala Lumpur, or K. L. The history revealed headache, prostration, and fever of five days, and upon examination, a tell-tale eschar in the right axilla with adjacent adenopathy. After examination, blood was taken for the routine laboratory evaluation of hemoglobin, leukocyte count, acute-phase serum for the Weil-Felix reaction, and injection of mice intraperitoneally for rickettsial isolation. A picture was taken of patient Osman in the hot midday sun (fig. 2).

A loading oral dose of 2 grams of chloromycetin using 250-milligram tablets was given with a subsequent schedule of one tablet every two hours until the tenth to twelfth day of illness. Joe had surmised that specific therapy should continue until emergence of *Proteus* OX K agglutinins which occurred usually late in the

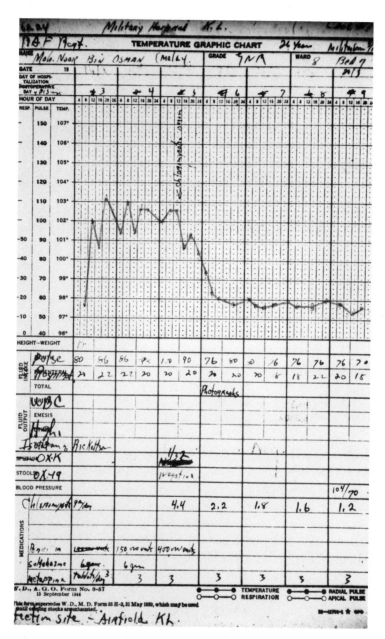

Figure 3. Original chart of first chloromycetin-treated scrub typhus patient, a twenty-six-year-old Malayan. Classic signs of fever, headache, macular rash, and eschar present on fifth febrile day. Treatment consisted of an initial oral dose of 2 grams and 250 milligrams every two hours until the twelfth day. Noticeable improvement within eighteen hours and afebrile twenty-four hours after instituting specific treatment. Diagnosis confirmed by isolation of R. orientalis *from blood and rise in* Proteus OX K *agglutinins. Rapid convalescence without relapse.*

second febrile week. By noon the next day, Osman was noticeably improved: less toxic in appearance, headache gone, and, twenty-four hours after beginning treatment, afebrile. Subsequently, the diagnosis of scrub typhus was confirmed by isolation of rickettsia and rise in titer of *Proteus* OX K agglutinins. Recovery was prompt and complete without relapse.

The second patient was Corporal Bebbington, of His Majesty's Forces, who was treated in the military hospital. Initially quite ill, he responded promptly within thirty hours and did not relapse (fig. 4).

A steady flow of suspect typhus patients in the civilian and military hospitals of K. L., in the nearby rubber estates, medical wards, and surrounding villages insured an adequate clinical trial. Among these ill patients was a hardy group of Gurkha soldiers who were treated in the military hospital. There was no simultaneously untreated control series. Patients thought to have scrub typhus were selected and treated consecutively. Of the first forty patients, thirty were confirmed as having scrub typhus. The additional ten included two with murine typhus, two with malaria, one with blackwater fever, two with leptospirosis, two with typhoid, to be described later, and two with GKW (God knows what). This represented a bedside clinical diagnostic batting average of seventy-five percent.

We experienced a striking example of the rapid spread of news. Lewthwaite received a telephone call from Stanley Pavillard, a prominent Singapore physician, whose patient, Mr. Smith, a banker, was desperately ill with typhus in its late stages. News had reached Singapore via a British Army Officer traveling by train from K. L. Familiar with the recovery of Corporal Bebbington, he related the miraculous event to another passenger, who was visiting the Smiths. Lewthwaite and I coerced Joe, in spite of his protestations, to broaden the area of patient selection and treat the banker in view of diplomatic amenities. The afternoon plane from Ipoh, which took me to Singapore, was strewn with flowers and carried an urn containing a portion of the ashes of Mahatma Ghandi. Approximately thirty thousand excited native Hindus met that plane. Pavillard cleverly extracted me from that huge throng and drove directly to the hospital. In spite of a domineering wife, who was a former nurse, impending vascular collapse, delirium, and a purplish exanthem, Banker Smith, case No. 9 in the series, recovered. This feat established beyond doubt that the antibiotic was remarkably effective at all stages.

Very early in the trials, Howard Florey, en route to London from Australia, stopped in K. L. to observe the trials. After personally witnessing the twenty-four-hour recovery of a scrub typhus patient and observing the clinical responses of the first few cases treated which had been displayed graphically, Florey remarked: "I'll buy it, you don't need statistical evidence."

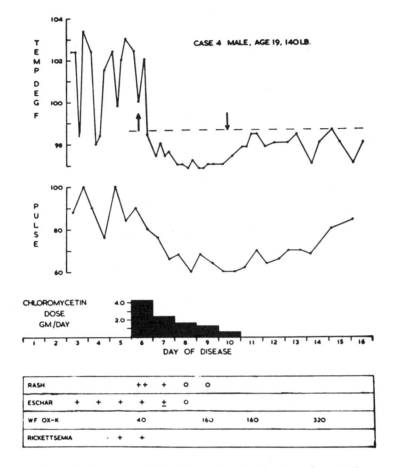

Figure 4. A very ill nineteen-year-old British corporal with classic signs of scrub typhus. Treatment initiated on the sixth day of illness. Systemic manifestations promptly abated and he was afebrile in twenty-four hours after beginning treatment. Diagnosis confirmed by rickettsial isolation and rise of Proteus OX K agglutinins. Reprinted from Science (Washington, DC), *1948, 108:160.*

Joe directed a tight laboratory program. Initial and convalescent blood specimens, daily temperature and pulse responses, and an audit of chloromycetin tablets were all duly recorded. Once he observed the pouring of serum from a tube of clotted blood. A quick retort: "Chum, hereafter the tube will be centrifuged and the serum pipetted." This admonition, with additional epithets, ended this practice.

Soon, it was clear that chloromycetin cured scrub typhus patients promptly. Based on this confidence, the therapeutic regimen was reduced to one day's treatment and even one 3-gram oral dose. All led to recovery without relapse provided treatment was initiated not earlier than the fifth day of illness. Relapses were later encountered in patients treated before the fifth febrile day. These clinical results provided a basis for understanding the difficulties encountered in the subsequent chemoprophylactic field trials.

On Saturday night, April 3, 1948, we were informed of two new febrile patients, Nos. 17 and 18 in the initial series, transported from a plantation ordinarily reliable as a source of scrub typhus patients (fig. 5). By candlelight, the brief clinical history and examination were completed and specimens obtained for laboratory evaluation. Both patients were toxic; neither had an eschar. In twenty-four hours, one patient was improved dramatically in keeping with the prior

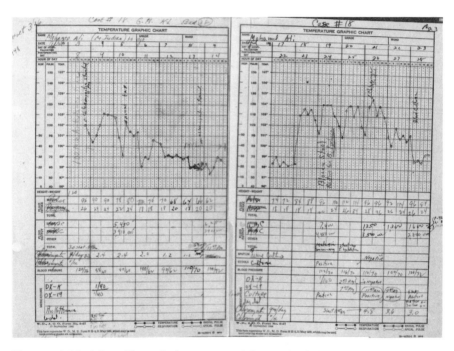

Figure 5. Original chart of first typhoid patient successfully treated with chloromycetin. This thirty-year-old Malayan was initially thought to have scrub typhus based on signs of fever, headache, prostration, and the fact that he came from a plantation where scrub typhus was very prevalent. Treatment started on the eighth day of illness. No noticeable improvement on the second day when diarrhea was present; the temperature remained elevated and he was toxic and apathetic. On the following day, he was clinically improved and on the third day following treatment, temperature had abated. When chloromycetin treatment was stopped, he had a relapse with a toxic psychosis which responded to additional chloromycetin treatment with full recovery. Diagnosis confirmed by isolation of Salmonella typhosa from blood, feces, and positive Widal reaction.

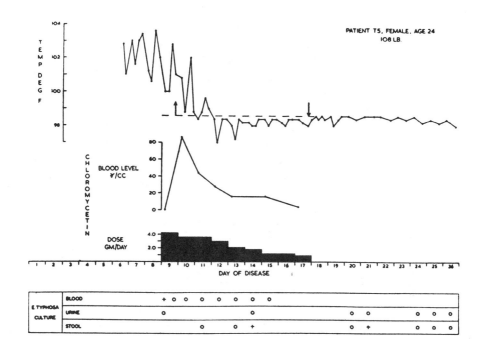

Figure 6. *Case T-5, one of the early selected typhoid fever patients treated with chloromycetin who became afebrile after three days of treatment. Recovery complete without relapse. Reprinted from* Annals of Internal Medicine, *1948, 29:131.*

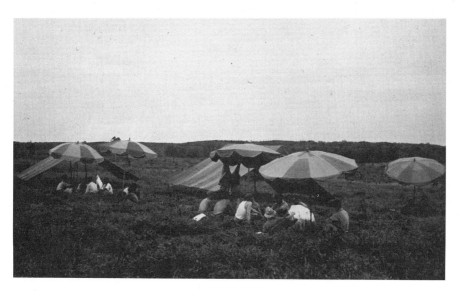

Figure 7. *Site of exposure of volunteers in a mite rickettsial-infested area at the Seaport Rubber Plantation near Kuala Lumpur.*

experience. The second patient, No. 18, was unchanged; he appeared toxic, apathetic with abdominal distress and diarrhea. Enteric fever was suspected. Since blood cultures were not included in our routine, an attempt was made to retrieve typhoid bacilli from the peritoneal exudate of mice inoculated with blood. The smear was not confirmatory but cultures of peritoneal exudate, and later specimens of the patient's blood, yielded typhoid bacilli. Joe was annoyed that precious chloromycetin tablets were being expended on a nonmission-oriented problem, but he relented. Within two days, some clinical improvement was apparent based

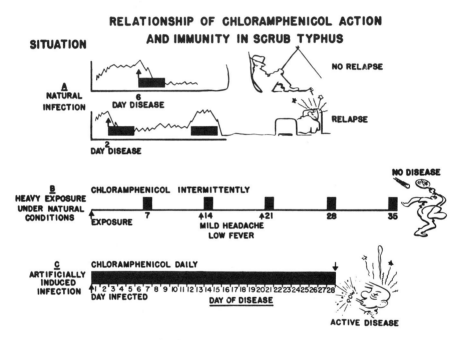

Figure 8. Scrub typhus chemoprophylaxis. Cartoon showing the various patterns of clinical response and relapse in induced scrub typhus volunteers given chloromycetin as a means of prevention. (A) Prompt response to chloromycetin treatment initiated on sixth day of illness, without relapse. Prompt response to chloromycetin treatment initiated on second day of illness with full relapse about eight days later. Relapse responded to retreatment. (B) Pattern in volunteers with heavy exposure to scrub typhus–infected mites under natural conditions. Intermittent single doses of chloromycetin given once weekly for five times resulted in no significant illness and no active infection after chemoprophylaxis stopped. (C) Volunteers injected subcutaneously with viable R. orientalis. Chloromycetin initiated at time of infection and continued daily for twenty-eight days. Active scrub typhus infection occurred about seven days after chemoprophylaxis stopped which indicated that the antibiotic was merely rickettsiostatic and immunity or resistance to infection had not developed. Reprinted from The Dynamics of Viral and Rickettsial Infections, *1955, McGraw-Hill Inc., New York, F. W. Hartman, F. L. Horsfall, and J. G. Kidd, eds.*

on bedside findings; defervescence occurred in about three days. Treatment was discontinued after five days of normal temperature; eight days later, I was greeted with a full-blown relapse and a toxic psychosis. The relapse responded to additional therapy.

The next several selected typhoid patients responded in less than four days and did not relapse (see fig. 6).

There was trouble ahead which caused a little familial unrest. Among the ten treated typhoid patients, two relapsed, one became temporarily psychotic, another developed gross hemorrhage which required transfusion, and one intestinal perforation with peritonitis and shock. Concerning this latter, very ill patient, selected for treatment on the seventeenth day, Joe remarked, "Why start treatment on such an ill patient. Do you want to ruin the series?" My retort that we ought to determine the true efficacy of the drug in typhoid gave little comfort. This patient's intestine perforated two days later; yet he and all other patients recovered. In spite of this inauspicious beginning, we were convinced of the therapeutic benefit and published the results based on ten typhoid patients.

After the obvious dramatic therapeutic response in scrub typhus patients, Joe directed the field chemoprophylactic studies. American, English, and Malayan volunteers were purposely exposed by sitting eight hours daily for ten days in a mite-ridden, typhus-infested area at the Seaport Rubber Plantation near K. L. (see fig. 7).

These human field trials, which extended for several years, revealed that clinical typhus infection could be suppressed by administering the antibiotic at intervals once every four or five days for about seven weeks. Shorter, intermittent regimens resulted in rickettsemia and clinical illness. Giving chloromycetin simultaneously at the first day of infection, daily for twenty-eight days, merely extended the incubation period; classic illness occurred seven days after stopping the drug (see fig. 8).

The therapeutic findings in patients and results of the field trials in volunteers demonstrated the rickettsiostatic properties of chloromycetin and established that resistance to infection bore a relationship to a sustained or sufficient intermittent antigenic stimulus. The field trials effectively demonstrated the immunologic relationships between host, microbe, and antibiotic, and provide essential guidelines of chemoprophylaxis based on active immunization. Charley Wisseman, Bennett Elisberg, Bob Traub, and others had a hand in the later field testing. Joe, himself a volunteer, developed a severe attack of typhus.

One night, Joe borrowed the "clinical" jeep which I alone used. He soon ran out of gas and after returning to the billet by foot, promptly awakened me for a lecture in automotive toilette. The breakfast atmosphere was rather chilly. That very day, at noon, after morning rounds, I parked in front of a Chinese cabinet maker's shop to check progress of a teakwood chest. The front door closed lightly and Joe entered and made a kind remark about my handsome chest. With great courage, he remarked, "I just ran out of gas with the other jeep, will you please push me back to the IMR." Perfect timing!

The initial venture to Kuala Lumpur ended in June 1948, with a total cost to our government of less than $50,000.

Joe's imaginative medical mission to Malaya was the forerunner of continued scientific collaboration between scientists of the Institute for Medical Research in Kuala Lumpur, WRAIR, and Maryland. The new therapeutic, epidemiologic, and preventive techniques resulting from this cooper-

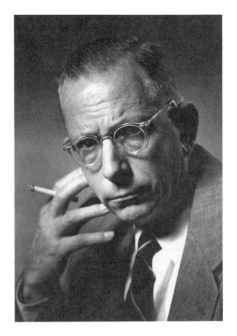

Figure 9. The late Joseph E. Smadel, ca. 1961. Photo courtesy of the author.

ative international program are a fitting tribute to this remarkably stimulating, vigorous, and talented medical scientist.

Now it is time to pay tribute to René Dubos, who was a giant among biologists and scholars. Just imagine a medical institute with persons like Dubos, Rivers, Avery, Dochez, MacLeod, Smadel, McCarty, Goodner, Francis, Horsfall, and many others, all at the same time.

René Dubos honored the University of Maryland on many occasions, not only by his presence but for his delivery of most stimulating lectures to faculty and students alike. He loved to lecture in our old Davidge Hall with its steeply tiered seats in a building which dates back to 1812. The audience was "always in his pocket" whether he was discussing medical science or philosophy. Once, because of extensive renovations, it was necessary for him to give his talk in a rather drab lecture hall. Afterward, he said, "Ted, if you do not put me in the old hall next time, I won't come." He returned several more times in the old setting; he was a favorite in Baltimore.

Once, René called to ask if he might use a quote which I had expressed on the occasion of a dinner meeting held in his honor after one of his lectures. The quote was really about a Bushman of the Kalahari Desert in Southwest Africa.

On being asked his age, the aged Bushman remarked, "I am as young as the most beautiful wish in my heart, and as old as all of the unfilled longings in my life."

This response also characterized René Dubos.

Bibliography

Bartz, Q. R. 1948. Isolation and characterization of chloromycetin. *Journal of Biological Chemistry.* 172:445.

Controulis, J., M. C. Rebstock, and H. M. Crooks, Jr. 1949. Chloramphenicol (chloromycetin). V. Synthesis. *Journal of the American Chemical Society.* 71:2463.

Ehrlich, J., Q. R. Bartz, R. M. Smith, D. A. Joslyn, and P. R. Burkholder. 1947. Chloromycetin, a new antibiotic from a soil actinomycete. *Science (Washington, DC).* 106:417.

Ehrlich, J., D. Gottlieb, P. R. Burkholder, L. E. Anderson, and T. G. Pridham. 1948. *Streptomyces venezuelae:* N. Sp. The source of chloromycetin. *Journal of Bacteriology.* 56:467.

Rebstock, M. C., H. M. Crooks, Jr., J. Controulis, and Q. R. Bartz. 1949. Chloramphenicol (chloromycetin). IV. Chemical studies. *Journal of the American Chemical Society.* 71:2458.

Smadel, J. E., and E. B. Jackson. 1947. Chloromycetin, an antibiotic with chemotherapeutic activity in experimental and viral infections. *Science (Washington, DC).* 106:418.

Smadel, J. E., T. E. Woodward, H. L. Ley, Jr., C. B. Philip, R. Traub, R. Lewthwaite, and S. R. Savoor. 1948. Chloromycetin in the treatment of scrub typhus. *Science (Washington, DC).* 108:160.

Smadel, J. E., R. Traub, H. L. Ley, Jr., C. B. Philip, T. E. Woodward, and R. Lewthwaite. 1949. Chloramphenicol (chloromycetin) in the chemoprophylaxis of scrub typhus (tsutsugamushi disease). II. Results with volunteers exposed in hyperendemic areas of scrub typhus. *American Journal of Hygiene.* 50:75.

Smith, R. M., D. A. Joslyn, O. M. Gruhzit, I. W. McLean, Jr., M. A. Prenner, and J. Ehrlich. 1948. Chloromycetin: biological studies. *Journal of Bacteriology.* 55:425.

Woodward, T. E., and C. L. Wisseman, Jr. 1958. Chloromycetin (chloramphenicol). In *Antibiotics Monographs No. 8.* New York: Medical Encyclopedia, Inc.

Woodward, T. E., J. E. Smadel, H. L. Ley, Jr., R. Green, and D. S. Mankikar. 1948. Preliminary report on the beneficial effect of chloromycetin in the treatment of typhoid fever. *Annals of Internal Medicine.* 29:131.

NEW REMEDIES
FOR AN ANCIENT
INFECTION:
ANTIBIOTICS AND
TUBERCULOSIS

George B. Mackaness

The October 1989 gathering created a unique opportunity for so many old friends to meet again and to kindle an echo of the excitement we felt in the opening decade of the antibiotic era. In preparing for the symposium I had the additional, if doubtful, pleasure of reading my doctoral thesis for the first time in thirty-seven years. I was surprised to find how much I had forgotten of the details that went into my tiny effort in pursuit of new remedies for ancient infections and of a deeper understanding of how to use those we already had. My recollections are so vivid that it is hard to believe we are celebrating the fiftieth anniversary of Dubos's discovery and development of gramicidin, the first clinically useful antibiotic.

Let me begin at the end of my story with an anecdote about my first encounter with René Dubos. I was very honored and excited to receive a letter from him in 1952. He said he was planning a trip to Oxford and wished to visit my laboratory. Upon inquiry, I was surprised to find that he had not informed anyone else of his intended visit. As a young graduate student, the thought of having to entertain so renowned a scientist filled me with apprehension; so I approached a very senior colleague with whom I was collaborating at the time, A. Q. Wells (see p. 20). AQ, as he was called, was a full six feet six inches of imposing dignity, an

President (Retired), The Squibb Institute for Medical Research. Studied with Howard Florey and worked on the tubercle bacillus and antibiosis. Later he pioneered studies in cell-mediated immunity.

aristocrat of immense wealth, and a diligent scientist. The Wells lived in the Manor House at Shipton-under-Wychwood. When AQ learned of Dubos's intended visit, he declared, "We must have a dinner party for him." I did not expect help on such a scale, but I was glad to transfer my social responsibilities to an acknowledged expert.

On the appointed Tuesday our visitor failed to appear; nor did he show up on Wednesday; or on Thursday morning for that matter. Since I had by then given up hope of seeing him at all, I set in motion an experiment that had been in preparation for a week and was scheduled to begin on the Thursday afternoon. No sooner were we under way than the door opened to reveal a huge man who all but filled the doorway. He was wearing a trench coat that made him seem even more massive. If I had ever seen Dubos or a likeness of him, I might have been spared the next few minutes of embarrassment. But thinking that the intruder was a salesman hawking his laboratory wares, I shot him a hostile glare and asked not to be interrupted. Before I could say anything more regrettable, my visitor, who was shifting uncomfortably from one foot to the other, announced that he was René Dubos. I can still feel the blush and remember the flustered welcome I gave while struggling to compose myself. The next few minutes were even more difficult, for I had to cancel an ongoing experiment without sacrificing all the work that had already gone into it, and to do so without being thought uncivil, or appearing indifferent to Dubos's presence. He seemed to understand and share my embarrassment.

The rest of Dubos's visit was an unqualified success, especially the dinner. The Manor House, its flagstone floors and sprinkling of oriental rugs, the right wines, and a retinue of servants at the table inspired Dubos to a stellar performance. He loved an attentive audience and was always prepared to contribute a lion's share to an evening's entertainment. This he did for us on that day which started so inauspiciously. Through the years, we enjoyed many more dinner parties enriched by his presence. My wife found special pleasure in debating with him the relative weights and shades of difference between English words with similar meanings. He loved English, the language he used for almost all of his vast technical, literary, and philosophical writings. Indeed, he seemed to take a perverse pride in the fact that he had published nothing in his native tongue until his final years. I can understand this sentiment in one who wrote and spoke English with such facility. His description of the Brooklyn Bridge in *The Torch of Life* (1962) bears witness to his skill with words.

Now I can return to the business of antibiosis, a field I entered inadvertently and to which, I confess at once, I contributed no new examples. I had arrived in Oxford from the British Postgraduate Medical School in 1948 with a view to taking a research degree under Howard Florey. Florey was an ideal mentor: strong willed, determined, and well informed. He was generous, not with praise but with advice, encouragement, wise guidance, and with his refusal to take any credit for the achievements of his students. When I asked him to share authorship of my first publication he said, in his curt manner of address, "That won't do you any good, Mackaness."

Florey set me to work initially on an uninspiring project that was aimed at determining whether mononuclear phagocytes are capable of responding to a chemotactic stimulus as had been demonstrated in the case of the more numerous polymorphonuclear phagocytes. Mononuclear phagocytes, the body's large scavenger cells, originate mainly from the bone marrow and circulate as a minor cellular constituent of blood where they are known as monocytes. These motile cells soon leave the blood to reside in the tissues until called into action for any one of a variety of purposes—to clear debris from traumatized tissue, to fight a localized infection, or to set up a barrier against invading tumor cells. Of special significance in the present context, the monocyte had been recognized for some time as the principal cell involved in fighting the tubercle bacillus. In fact, most of the cells in the inflammatory reaction to a focus of proliferating tubercle bacilli are monocytes which have arrived there from the blood. These monocytes undergo striking changes in morphology and metabolic activity as they adapt to their role of defense against such a formidable foe. Unfortunately, the tubercle bacillus is also an adaptor: it has learned to live and multiply within the very cells that the body relies upon for its primary defenses. Despite this, the immunity developed against the tubercle bacillus is usually successful; but that is another story.

While it was obviously important to know from direct observation whether monocytes are capable of moving deliberately towards the objective source of a chemotactic substance such as a collection of tubercle bacilli, the larger questions of what they do after arriving at an infective focus, why their mission sometimes fails, and what can be done to help them, were issues of greater interest to me. But as a novice I felt more comfortable with Florey's simpler, better-defined project for my maiden excursion into investigative biology. For this I needed only a source of monocytes and an ability to follow the techniques that others had already used to show that polymorphs move toward a chemotactic target like moths to a candle. I was soon on the trail, for a predecessor of mine at the Trudeau Sanatorium, Leroy Gardner, had published a paper in 1929 (1) showing that the free fluid in the peritoneal cavity of guinea pigs contains large numbers of normal-looking monocytes. Three or four years later, Stuart Mudd and his colleagues (2) showed how this population of monocytes could be enormously enriched by instilling mineral oil into the peritoneal cavity several days before harvesting its

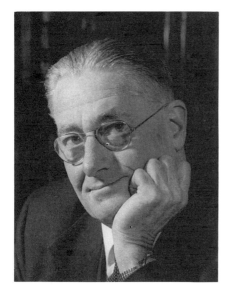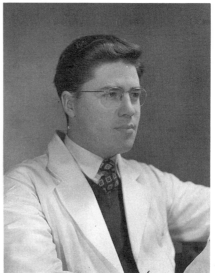

Howard Florey (left) *and his graduate student George Mackaness* (right), *University of Oxford, around 1950. Courtesy of the Sir William Dunn School of Pathology.*

cellular contents. In my hands over a period of years the average number of cells recovered from rabbits so treated was 280 million, 90% of which were unequivocal monocytes.

With an abundant source of monocytes as a starting point, and the help and advice of many people in the laboratories, some of them fellow doctoral students, I learned how to keep them under cultural conditions in vitro, how to observe and photograph them under living conditions, and many other ancillary techniques. In a relatively short time I had obtained crude evidence that monocytes behaved much as polymorphs did toward a chemotactic stimulus. Obviously, I would have to demonstrate the validity of this finding by more elegant and convincing methods. To add interest to the project, however, my private thoughts and experimental ambitions had begun to embrace a phenomenon of greater potential importance.

In 1927, Murray, Webb, and Swan (3) encountered a lethal infection in laboratory rabbits which was associated with a massive increase in the number of monocytes in circulation. The authors isolated an unknown microorganism from the infected animals and showed that it could reproduce the disease in normal rabbits. They called it *Bacillus monocytogenes*. This organism, which is also pathogenic for man, is now known as *Listeria monocytogenes*. I fell to wondering how it caused such a massive outpouring of young monocytes. One possibility was by releasing a substance that causes monocytes or their precursors to replicate. Since the monocyte was believed to be crucial to an effective defense against tuberculosis, a monocytogenic substance might have therapeutic applications. I set out with Florey's approval to explore this possibility. I had reached the stage of showing that *L. monocytogenes*, dead or alive, did not cause monocytes to grow in tissue culture, but that the dead organism caused a brisk monocytosis when injected intravenously into rabbits. Moreover, cell fragments and cell-free extracts of dead *Listeria* were also monocytogenic. Attempts to extract the active substance had just begun when we received a visit from Macfarlane Burnet. Florey accompanied him to my laboratory and they both listened patiently till the end of my story. At this point, Burnet turned to Florey and said, "I'd take him off that project, Florey. Neville Stanley has just submitted a paper to *The Australian Journal of Biology and Experimental Science* [of which Burnet was Editor-in-Chief] describing a monocytogenic phospholipid that he extracted from *Listeria monocytogenes*." A few days later, Florey came to see me with a new project.

In time, I came to realize that it had always been Florey's intention to broaden the scope of my research. Several people at the Dunn School had begun working on a new antibiotic called micrococcin. Florey's interest in micrococcin rested on two facts: it had some inhibitory activity against the tubercle bacillus; and it was very sparingly soluble in water, so much so that it could not be administered in free solution in amounts sufficient to demonstrate an antituberculous effect in infected mice and guinea pigs. Florey, speculating on the merits of reducing micrococcin to a fine powder that could be administered intravenously as an aqueous suspension, had enlisted Norman Heatley to make a suitable preparation. Neil Markham, a fellow D.Phil. student from New Zealand, was given the task of finding out whether micrococcin particles in the blood could penetrate to tubercle bacilli living and multiplying in the cellular accumulations known as tubercles. As I have mentioned, these characteristic lesions which gave their name to the disease are made up predominantly of physiologically modified monocytes.

Florey's new research proposal for me was disclosed in the following exchanges. "Mackaness, you've got monocytes in culture." "Yes sir." "Could you infect them with tubercle bacilli, make them ingest particles of micrococcin, and then see whether the ingested antibiotic can prevent the tubercle bacilli from multiplying when the monocyte cultures are incubated?"

When I allowed that this might be technically feasible, Florey enlarged on his notion that monocytes could perhaps be "fortified" with particles of a relatively insoluble antibiotic. This was probably the first mention of the possibility that poorly soluble antibiotics might be administered in depot form to increase their duration of action, a principle that was later applied successfully to penicillin. In the case of tuberculosis, Florey's notion had special appeal in that the depot of antibiotic would be distributed diffusely through the body, yet be concentrated within the cells that become the habitat of invading tubercle bacilli. This was Florey's pet project for a year or two.

At first I thought that the proposed experiments would be relatively easy to perform, but I soon learned that no one had ever attempted to measure the growth and death of intracellular organisms in tissue culture. One of the most critical requirements for work of this type was a method for determining the number of viable organisms in any given location. Until shortly before I began work on my new project, this could not be done with tubercle bacilli because of their high content of waxes which made them intensely hydrophobic. The unwettable bacilli adhere tenaciously to each other, forming tangled skeins that float on the surface of simple aqueous culture media. The resulting mass of bacilli resist the fiercest efforts to extricate even a few individual bacilli for experimental purposes. Fortunately, Dubos, at The Rockefeller Institute in New York, needed a highly dispersed suspension of tubercle bacilli and a reliable method of determining how many living tubercle bacilli it contained, so that he could inoculate animals with known numbers of them. He suggested to his colleague Bernard Davis how this might be done with the aid of a detergent. Bernie rendered the idea into a practical culture medium in which most strains of the tubercle bacillus would grow in a highly dispersed state from which single-celled suspensions could be readily prepared. The Davis-Dubos media (4), liquid and solid, became indispensable tools to all who would work quantitatively with the tubercle bacillus (see page 92). Without them I would not have been able to reach the goal that Florey had set for me, because they enabled me to infect monocytes with a discrete number of tubercle bacilli and determine whether the bacilli in cells were alive or had succumbed to an antibiotic or combination of antibiotics.

In the coming months, I learned to infect monocytes with known numbers of various strains of tubercle bacilli, to observe them microscopically in the company of rabbit monocytes, to maintain the cells under constant observation in specially designed culture chambers, and to determine the fate of the organisms under a variety of experimental conditions. To reach this stage of technical competence, it took me an embarrassing eighteen months. Once there, however, results came quickly; but the answer to my part of the micrococcin story was profoundly disappointing. Though clearly visible in the cytoplasm of every monocyte by virtue of its strong blue fluorescence in ultraviolet light, the micrococcin served to inhibit the growth of bacilli in cells for only a few days. Subsequent observations showed that the bacilli had become tolerant of the antibiotic.

By the time I had reached this conclusion, Neil Markham had uncovered an equally discouraging fact: cells harboring tubercle bacilli in the inner parts of a tubercle were not accessible to particulate material administered through the blood stream (5). In light of this and my own observations, it was not surprising to find that micrococcin could not stop a tuberculous infection from progressing to a fatal outcome. But Florey was not yet ready to abandon micrococcin. His next move was to call for a colloidal solution of the antibiotic in the hope that in this form it would behave like the colloidal dyes which had been used so successfully in living animals to stain cells of the reticuloendothelial system, to which the monocyte belongs. The technical problem of making a colloidal solution of micrococcin was solved by Norman Heatley. As a dispersing agent, Heatley chose Triton WR1339, which belonged to a newly discovered chemical series known as polyoxyethylene ethers. Although the good-looking, slightly viscous colloidal solution of micrococcin proved to be no more effective than powdered micrococcin, I mention these additional studies with micrococcin because Triton WR1339 was found to possess some very interesting properties.

Cornforth et al. (6) had shown that some surface-active agents, including the polyoxyethylene ethers, had antituberculous activity in vivo even though they actually facilitated growth of virulent tubercle bacilli in vitro. After learning from me that Triton had no effect on tubercle bacilli living in monocytes maintained in its presence, Dick Rees suggested that I should test monocytes obtained from rabbits that had been injected repeatedly with the detergent. Upon doing this, I was surprised to find that the monocytes from Triton-treated animals had undergone a profound functional change which made them immune to challenge with tubercle bacilli in tissue culture. Not only were tubercle bacilli unable to multiply in monocytes from Triton-treated rabbits, but bacilli of some strains actually disappeared from the cytoplasm after a few days in culture. It is now suspected that the detergent, which is known to enter monocytes, acts to wet the bacilli and render them susceptible to the phagocytes' normal antimicrobial and digestive mechanisms. It is regrettable, therefore, that Triton WR1339 and other surface-active agents cause severe disturbances of fat metabolism and are prohibitively toxic.

Having two more or less negative results to my credit, I was anxious to test other antituberculous drugs in the hope of better luck. Since I had by now a good grip on the technique, it was not long before I had tested all seven of those available at that time. The results, summarized in Table I (adapted from references 7 and 8), were revealing. Paraaminosalicylic acid, which performed better than micrococcin against experimental infections in animals without actually curing them, was even less effective than micrococcin against intracellular tubercle

Table I.   Drug activities against extra- and intracellular tubercle bacilli.

| | Lowest inhibitory concentration | |
	Extracellular	Intracellular
	μg/ml	*μg/ml*
Paraaminosalicylic acid	1.56	1.56
Streptomycin	0.60	10.00–25.00
Terramycin	12.50	12.50
Neomycin	1.56	25.00
Viomycin	6.25	100.00
Nisin	5.00	No activity
Isoniazid	0.03	0.05

Adapted from references 7 and 8.

bacilli. In spite of only modest potency and its tendency to cause severe nausea, paraaminosalicylic acid is still in use today for reasons I shall discuss later.

Streptomycin was the first really effective chemotherapeutic agent against tuberculosis. It was discovered by Schatz, Bougie, and Waksman (9) in 1944, but did not become widely available until 1947. Even in those days, when significant advances in treatment for infectious diseases were so urgently needed and questions of safety and efficacy were treated less rigorously than nowadays, years always intervened between discovery and availability of significant new drugs. This makes it all the more remarkable that gramicidin and penicillin were brought to the clinic almost as quickly as streptomycin was. Though the latter was strongly bactericidal at low concentrations, Steenken and Pratt (10) had found that maximum tolerated doses of streptomycin were unable to kill tubercle bacilli in the tissues of experimentally infected animals until they had become tuberculin sensitive, implying the acquisition of resistance to the infection. And even then the drug was unable to halt the progress of infection completely. This was not due to development of resistance, though this happened quite quickly during treatment with streptomycin. The fundamental problem was found to lie in the drug's inability to reach bactericidal concentrations in the cytoplasm of infected cells. The tissue culture studies showed clearly that infected monocytes continued to harbor living tubercle bacilli even when the drug concentration in the culture medium was far higher than could be safely achieved in the body. This, and the rapid emergence of drug resistance, accounted for the fact that streptomycin was less effective clinically than its microbicidal potency would have predicted.

Unfortunately, none of the other drugs available in 1951 was any better than streptomycin. Among them was terramycin, which was alone in demonstrating that antibiotics could be equally active against intra- and extracellular tubercle bacilli. Terramycin, however, was not a potent drug and its action was strictly bacteriostatic. It played no part in the conquest of tuberculosis. This left clinicians with just two drugs with which to battle the tubercle bacillus. Fortunately, it was quickly established that streptomycin and paraaminosalicylic acid, acting together, were able to curtail the emergence of drug resistance. But even in combination they could not effect a speedy cure, though they did significantly reduce the death rate from tuberculosis.

Come 1952! I had just begun to write my thesis and was impatient to be back in the lab when an unexpected package came by mail. It contained a number of vials, each holding a small sample of six different compounds that were said to have some activity against the tubercle bacillus. They had been sent to me by Herts Pharmaceuticals Ltd., a small and newly established company with whom Florey had discussed the possibility of synthesizing some insoluble thiosemicarbazides for his pet project. That was before it had fallen from grace with the discovery that particulate antibiotics were unlikely to work in tuberculosis, regardless of potency. Five of the vials contained thiosemicarbazides. The sixth contained "a 10-gram sample of the new antituberculous drug that was announced last week in *The New York Times*." So read the handwritten note that accompanied the package. It seems that an officer of Herts Pharmaceuticals happened to be in New York and to have read a newspaper account of the response to a new drug being used in severely ill tuberculous patients at the Bellevue Hospital. The drug was identified as isonicotinic acid hydrazide, or isoniazid as it became known officially. This news was telephoned to the home office in London on the same Friday. By Monday morning enough isoniazid had been made to send me a generous sample that arrived two days later.

I learned subsequently from Walsh McDermott that he had been approached independently by the directors of research at Squibb and at Hoffman La Roche, each asking him to organize a clinical trial on a promising new drug for tuberculosis. So similar were their claims that McDermott, the influential editor of the *American Review of Tuberculosis*, suspected that each was speaking of the same compound and that one of them must have been supplying the drug to clinicians at Bellevue Hospital. So he called them together for discussions. It was fortunate, perhaps, that isonicotinic acid had first been synthesized in 1929, so there could be no question of either company obtaining patent rights for their discovery. Nonetheless, both companies agreed to share in underwriting the clinical trials that were promptly undertaken on a large scale.

It was fortunate for me that the early investigation of isoniazid had been conducted in great secrecy, and also that Herts Pharmaceuticals had sent me some of it to test before anyone outside the two drug houses knew anything of its existence. Within four weeks I had found that isoniazid was powerfully and equally bactericidal for both intra- and extracellular tubercle bacilli. It combined well with streptomycin to produce an even more rapid and potent bactericidal effect. When tested in tissue culture it produced complete sterilization of infected monocytes at drug concentrations that were achievable in man. In short, it brought a dramatic change in outlook for those seeking to improve the management of tuberculosis. In my test system it behaved in a way that lent credence to the glowing newspaper reports of its apparent clinical efficacy.

Although other good drugs have been added to the list (there are now eleven drugs in current use for the treatment of tuberculosis), isoniazid is still the one most commonly used. To convey a sense of how important it was in the battle against tuberculosis, I can tell you that five years after the introduction of streptomycin no reduction had occurred in the number of hospital beds being occupied by tuberculous patients in the United States. Five years after the discovery of isoniazid, eighty percent of the beds available in TB hospitals were unoccupied, and many sanatoria had closed their doors. A famous one was destined to become a jail; and a nearby neighbor became a research institute in the field of immunology. It would be wrong, however, to attribute all of this progress to isoniazid. No one drug by itself could have produced cure rates as spectacular as those being achieved by 1957. The real breakthrough in the management of tuberculosis came from the experiments and astute observations of the many clinicians, microbiologists, and pathologists whose work collectively established that the biggest barrier to a cure for tuberculosis was the development of drug resistance; and that simultaneous administration of two or more drugs that did not actively antagonize each other (as some drug combinations do) could be relied upon to prevent the emergence of drug resistance in most patients. The application of this therapeutic principle has changed the face of the disease that Dubos described so vividly in *The White Plague* (1952). Sad to say, tuberculosis is still with us and is almost as devastating in some countries as it ever was. The problem now is not the unavailability of effective treatment, but the inability of health services to afford the costs involved in finding and treating all of the afflicted millions.

In reflecting on all of this, I find it exciting to recognize that man usually meets with a measure of success when he turns his mind to the solution of a problem. Whether he will always be successful in finding ways of controlling all of the serious diseases that afflict him remains to be seen. Our society faces a present threat from AIDS. Few can be heard to say with confidence that this disease will soon be treatable or preventable. There is good reason, however, to expect that the level of research effort being deployed against the human immuno-deficiency virus will teach us vastly more about the immunology of virus infections and bring us an array of antiviral drugs that are more effective and more specific than any we have today. I am also optimistic that we will learn to treat or prevent most of the common, costly, and debilitating diseases attributable to atherosclerosis. But I fear that in this case the best measures, such as dietary discipline, will be unacceptable to many who would prefer to suffer the consequences than endure the sacrifices needed to avoid the heart attacks, the strokes, or the kidney failures that might or might not overtake them.

I would like to end this reminiscence with another anecdote. The incident occurred when I was a professorial fellow in the Department of Experimental Pathology at the Australian National University in Canberra, an institution that was the outcome of Florey's recommendations in 1947 to John Curtin, the Australian Prime Minister. Florey happened to be visiting the John Curtin School of Medical Research at the ANU in 1959 when I was about to take a sabbatical leave with René Dubos at The Rockefeller University. I told Florey of my impending visit to work with Dubos. His face lit up with evident pleasure, pleasure of a sort I had seen expressed once before. On that occasion, Florey had come to tell me that Alexander Fleming had called him for permission to invite me to take part in a symposium in Paris that he was organizing. I suppose it was British etiquette that required an approach to a graduate student by way of his mentor. Be that as it may, it was Florey's comment that mattered: "I'm really delighted to think that one of my students has received an invitation like this from Fleming. You know, Mackaness, some people seem to believe there is animosity between Fleming and me. I suppose they think there should be. But Fleming and I are good friends, though we seldom have contact these days." Florey's remark upon learning that I was going to work with Dubos evoked a similar expression of sentiment that I relate in his own words. "How delightful. One great sorrow I have was that Dubos was not recognized independently for a Nobel Prize. He did set the stage; he taught us how to find antibiotics; and I think he earned it."

I think many of us believe so too.

References

1. Gardner, L. U. 1929. Differential cell counts of the peritoneal fluid from the normal guinea pig. *Proceedings of the Society for Experimental Biology and Medicine.* 26:690.

2. Lucke, B., M. Strumia, S. Mudd, M. McCutcheon, and E. B. H. Mudd. 1933. On the comparative phagocytic activity of macrophage and polymorphonuclear leucocyte. *Journal of Immunology.* 24:455.

3. Murray, E. G. D., R. A. Webb, and M. B. R. Swan. 1926. A disease of rabbits characterised by a large mononuclear leucocytosis, caused by a hitherto undescribed bacillus, *Bacterium monocytogenes. Journal of Pathology and Bacteriology.* 29:407.

4. Dubos, R. J., and B. D. Davis. 1946. Factors affecting the growth of tubercle bacilli in liquid media. *Journal of Experimental Medicine.* 83:409.

5. Markam, N. P., N. G. Heatley, A. G. Sanders, and H. W. Florey. 1951. The behaviour in vivo of particulate micrococcin. *British Journal of Experimental Pathology.* 32:136.

6. Cornforth, J. W., P. D'A. Hart, R. J. W. Rees, and J. A. Stock. 1951. Antituberculous effect of certain surface-active polyoxyethylene ethers in mice. *Nature (London).* 168:150.

7. Mackaness, G. B. 1952. The action of drugs on intracellular tubercle bacilli. *Journal of Pathology and Bacteriology.* 64:429.

8. Mackaness, G. B., and N. Smith. 1952. The action of isoniazid (isonicotinic acid hydrazide) on intracellular tubercle bacilli. *American Review of Tuberculosis and Pulmonary Diseases.* 66:125.

9. Schatz, A., E. Bougie, and S. A. Waksman. 1944. Streptomycin, a substance exhibiting antibiotic activity against gram-positive and gram-negative bacteria. *Proceedings of the Society for Experimental Biology and Medicine.* 55:66.

10. Steenken, W., Jr., and P. C. Pratt. 1949. Streptomycin in experimental tuberculosis. *American Review of Tuberculosis and Pulmonary Diseases.* 59:664.

TWO PERSPECTIVES: ON RENÉ DUBOS, AND ON ANTIBIOTIC ACTIONS

Bernard D. Davis

Because René Dubos had an enormously beneficial influence on my own career, I particularly appreciate this opportunity to pay homage to him. In doing so I will pursue both suggestions in the invitation: to discuss my own experiences in working with him, but also to write under a broader title: Perspectives on Antibiotics. In pursuing the first topic I will also emphasize the difference in research style between Dubos and another pioneer in antibiotic research, his teacher Selman Waksman. And in discussing antibiotic action I will focus on my own research, which has led to a general conclusion that I know would have interested Dubos: The search for a single key action, which has been taken for granted in antibiotic research, can be misleading, as it has turned out to be for one major group, the aminoglycosides.

In considering the qualities that made Dubos so influential, among scientists and later to a wider public, I will also compare critically his talents as a critic and as an experimenter. I am sure this approach is what he would expect of me. For during the year that I spent in his laboratory we argued incessantly and intensely about all kinds of problems, scientific and social. I was the naive, idealistic young American, seeking absolute truths and social perfection, while he was the worldly

Adele Lehman Professor of Bacterial Physiology Emeritus, Harvard Medical School. Collaborated with René Dubos in the mid-1940s on tuberculosis research. Used antimicrobial agents to uncover basic tenets of bacterial physiology and genetics; explained mode of action of streptomycin.

European, seeing subtle complexities in every problem. We were rather like Herr Settembrini and Herr Naphta in *The Magic Mountain.*

First: how I got to Dubos's laboratory. During my four years as a medical student at Harvard I had done research part-time with E. J. Cohn, in one of the few laboratories in the world then devoted to protein chemistry. Hence when I served in the United States Public Health Service (USPHS) during World War II I was assigned to war projects under two outstanding immunologists, Elvin Kabat and Jules Freund. At the end of the war I accepted the invitation from the newly formed Tuberculosis Control Division of the USPHS to set up a laboratory to explore whatever aspects of tuberculosis seemed interesting. In view of the subsequently expanded role of the USPHS in biomedical science it may be of interest to note Cohn's annoyance that I would remain in such an obscure research organization, rather than returning to a university!

Immunology had not yet reached the stage where its complex phenomena could be translated into mechanisms, and I did not feel much attraction to the field. I decided instead to pursue microbiological aspects of the problem of tuberculosis—though in medical school I had also been bored by bacteriology, for the same reason. I now needed training in research in this field, and Dubos's laboratory looked to be the most exciting place. It did indeed prove to be very exciting.

Dubos had just devised a simple medium in which the waxy tubercle bacillus grew in a somewhat dispersed manner rather than in the usual large clumps. The medium contained the non-ionic detergent Tween 80, and also bovine serum albumin. With my background in protein chemistry I naturally studied the function of the albumin. I had already found, while an intern at Johns Hopkins Hospital, that it binds sulfonamide drugs; and I now found that it bound traces of fatty acids, coming not only from residual soap on the glassware but also from slow hydrolysis of the Tween during the weeks of incubation; the fatty acids were strongly inhibitory to the tubercle bacillus (1). This finding emphasized that a growth factor for bacteria might promote growth by providing protection, without serving as a nutrient.

Another implication was that the accepted role of albumin in mammalian blood, in supporting colloid osmotic pressure, was only part of its function (2). In fact, I also found traces of free fatty acids in human serum (3), which were evidently rendered nontoxic by the albumin. But I later realized that my publication of such an isolated finding as an aside in a methods paper, without a followup, had been worthless. Dubos used to say that a scientific paper should never try to make more than one point. The free fatty acid fraction in serum became recognized only after its rediscovery, decades later, in studies that also established its significance as a rapidly turning-over fraction in lipid metabolism.

My choice of Dubos's laboratory had been based largely on reading his recently published volume, *The Bacterial Cell*. As noted by Joshua Lederberg in the Introduction, this was a remarkably valuable book, summing up critically all the solid things we knew about bacteria, just before the field was revolutionized by the emergence of bacterial genetics. Dubos, of course, immediately recognized the importance of this new development. He frequently discussed, with great admiration, the work of Oswald Avery, which launched bacterial as well as molecular genetics; and he closed his own paper at the 1946 Cold Spring Harbor Symposium with a statement that illustrates his literary bent as well as his appreciation of the science: "With this discovery [of transformation by DNA] bacterial variation passes from the collector's box of the naturalist to the sophisticated atmosphere of the biochemistry laboratory. One may wonder whether the geneticist will not arrive too late to introduce his jargon into bacteriology." He was almost right: what bacterial geneticists subsequently did was not so much avoid classical jargon as create their own.

The beginning of another major development in microbiology, the analysis of enzyme induction, reached the laboratory while I was there, in the form of Jacques Monod's Ph.D. thesis on diauxie, which initiated his monumental work on gene regulation. I recall the excitement that this paper generated, and Dubos's great enthusiasm. He himself had written a review on bacterial adaptation in 1940 (4), but it missed the fundamental distinction between genotypic and phenotypic adaptation. He now recognized that this young student in Paris had put his finger on something very clear and important in this area. I suspect that its French origin added an extra dimension to his enthusiasm, for while he was thoroughly adapted to this country René Dubos retained a natural pride in French culture.

Dubos was then finishing his biography of Louis Pasteur (5), and he invited me to read the manuscript. I could not escape the feeling that Louis Pasteur must have been very much a model for him: both liked to deal with problems that combined intellectual and practical challenges, and both had a talent for dramatizing their work. But though Dubos was a dedicated experimenter, I felt that he did not have quite Pasteur's flair for the key experiment that would convincingly establish a profound principle, in one problem after another. On the other hand, Dubos had stronger literary, poetic, and philosophical interests and talents; his book on Pasteur, and his comments in conversation on other scientific developments, showed great critical acuity and sense of significance.

Since this volume commemorates the importance of Dubos's contribution to the development of antibiotic research, I now feel slightly uncomfortable in noting that at the time when I was there his evaluation of that field was rather negative. I recall that we discussed several times his earlier experience in the

Waksman laboratory, and then gramicidin and its disappointing toxicity. Rollin Hotchkiss mentioned that a few years earlier Dubos had expressed skepticism about penicillin because of its reported instability, but then it proved to be stable when Ernst Chain purified it. During my stay, in 1944 or 1945, Dubos further expressed doubt that any antibiotic was likely to turn up again with the fortunate nontoxicity of penicillin; hence the major future advances against infectious disease would have to arise from increased understanding of the organisms and the host defenses. (Waksman had announced streptomycin in 1944, but its clinical value had not yet been established—and it is, in fact, quite toxic compared with penicillin.)

Dubos's prediction was partly right, and his view might have helped to dispel the growing, widespread misconception that antibiotics would solve all problems of infectious disease. But his experience with gramicidin clearly had made him too bearish on antibiotics. Yet, if I may borrow from the title of one of his books, *So Human an Animal*, it was quite human to have become skeptical after having to abandon a product that seemed so promising but then turned out to be too toxic for systemic use.

To pursue the psychology of the search for antibiotics a bit further, let me contrast Dubos's attitude or style with that of Waksman, which Hotchkiss has already discussed in some detail. I would reinforce the picture of Waksman as primarily a natural historian of the soil, cataloging the microorganisms found there, and focusing on their taxonomy and their ecological effects. He was not a person with the intellectual restlessness that characterized Dubos. But perhaps for that very reason, he was more patient with a kind of search that had to survive several dead ends before yielding a product with the selective toxicity necessary for chemotherapy. Conversely, it would not have been natural for Dubos, always seeking creative new approaches to problems, to have adopted that kind of career.

As you have heard, the first antibiotic that Waksman isolated, actinomycin, was too toxic for use as an antimicrobial (though it later was found to be useful in cancer chemotherapy, where the margin of safety is less stringent). But the important point is that he persisted, and after encountering several other toxic antibiotics he finally hit streptomycin. This discovery, of the first effective antimicrobial agent against the dread scourge of tuberculosis, was rewarded with a Nobel Prize.

I would like to offer a somewhat different view of Waksman's achievement. Many years later, when I had the occasion to make some remarks at his funeral in Woods Hole, I was struck by the thought that his really important discovery was not streptomycin: it was the principle that a patient, systematic search for useful antibiotics will eventually pay off. With this discovery, the search for antibiotics took off in industry, and the result has been several thousand new compounds, among which roughly a hundred are useful. Moreover, their uses have been extended to areas other than antimicrobial action—for example, cyclosporin as a suppressor of autoimmune responses to organ transplants.

If there is any general moral here, it is the obvious one that different aspects of science benefit from different personalities and styles. And if this were an earlier era, before the recent extensive involvement of molecular biologists in biotechnology, one might be tempted to adjure biologists to change the snobbish attitude that most of us then felt toward applied aspects of our field.

Let me now spend a moment on a side issue that may have some historical interest: the attitudes of microbiologists toward the dangers in the laboratory, at the time when I worked with Dubos. Historically, most researchers who worked on the tubercle bacillus got started while they were convalescing in a sanatorium and hence had partial immunity, reflected in their tuberculin-positive state. Tuberculin-negative persons are more susceptible to the initial infection. I was tuberculin negative when I was invited to set up a tuberculosis research laboratory, but it did not enter my mind that my lack of any specific immunity to the organism might be a reason to refuse. On the contrary, there was a strong medical tradition that laboratory investigators of infectious disease, like physicians in epidemics, must accept the risk of being exposed to dangerous agents as part of the job.

Actually, it was more than willingness to accept a necessary risk. There was a rather "macho" attitude on the subject—just as in organic chemistry, where graduate students were sometimes dismissed, in the same era, because they objected to excessive exposure to organic solvents. And in the course of the history of microbiology over 400 deaths have been recorded from infections acquired in the laboratory (and perhaps quite a few not recorded). Yet in the work on biological warfare in Fort Detrick in World War II, involving highly virulent pathogens, negative-pressure hoods were developed and there were very few infections. However, in Dubos's laboratory we used hoods with ultraviolet radiation but no air flow, and we actually used unplugged pipettes to deal with virulent tubercle bacilli—I once got a mouthful of a culture. As a present frequent defender of science against those who dwell on highly hypothetical dangers, I am tempted to suggest that on the other side, the autonomy of science can sometimes benefit from outside encouragement of prudence.

Anyhow, I did develop clinical tuberculosis, halfway through my year in that laboratory, but I was fortunate in having a minimal, very peripheral lesion, which presented itself as a spontaneous pneumothorax. After a year of bedrest had proved ineffective the lesion was finally eliminated by excision of the infected

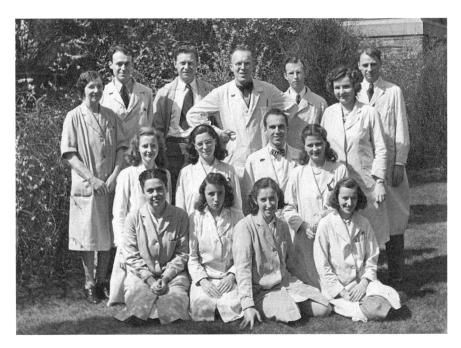

René Dubos's laboratory group at The Rockefeller Institute for Medical Research in 1946. (Rear, left to right) Jane Kramer, Bernard D. Davis, Alfred Marshak, René Dubos, Merrill Chase, Cynthia Pierce (now Chase), and Rollin Hotchkiss. (Center row, left to right) Margaret Brophy, Harlean Cort, Gardner Middlebrook, and Anne Christiansen. (Front, left to right) Jane Buckalew, unknown, Hannah Schott-lander, and Mary Andrews. Photo courtesy of the author.

tissue. (I subsequently discovered that I had become a rare if not unique object: a person who reverted to tuberculin negative without the benefit of chemotherapy, presumably because the organism never reached lymph nodes where it could be sequestered for the host's lifetime.)

In a curious way, this infection turned out to be a boon. There is an extensive and romantic literature, discussed by Dubos and his wife Jean in their book *The White Plague* (1952), claiming that tuberculosis tends to afflict creative people. I doubt that the bacillus has any basis for such selectivity in its choice of victims. On the other hand, its major impact has been on young adults, and the traditional treatment gave the victims a prolonged opportunity to suspend their daily routines and engage in reading and reflection. The lucky survivors may thus have had a chance to improve their perspective on their goals and hence sometimes to become more creative.

In my case, this period of enforced rest was in a sense an early sabbatical, at a stage in my life when I had finished my training and was about to set up an independent laboratory. In my reading during that year what impressed me most was a review by George Beadle on "biochemical" mutants of the mold *Neurospora* (6), a class (which I later named auxotrophic) that is blocked in the synthesis of some essential metabolite. This area of research attracted me at once, because it was close to the trunk of the biological tree and not on a peripheral twig. Though I had not studied genetics, and I had no plans for getting into this field, the seed persisted; and as we shall see, it eventually blossomed.

After a further period in Dubos's laboratory, following recovery from the operation and the disease, in 1947 I set up a tuberculosis research laboratory for the USPHS, in a New York City Health Center on East 69th Street. This space, conveniently close to The Rockefeller Institute, had been lent by the city to Cornell University Medical College to house its Department of Preventive Medicine, whose chairman, Wilson Smilley, lent it to the USPHS. I chose to work on a problem indirectly related to tuberculosis, the mechanism of action of streptomycin (which could be studied in *Escherichia coli*). In retrospect, I suspect that my infection may have given me an aversion to further work on the tubercle bacillus, and certainly to inviting nonimmune scientists to do so.

By then the fundamental action of penicillin was understood, since its lysis of the cell implied an action on the cell envelope, and the work of J. T. Park and J. L. Strominger identified its site of action as the cross-linking reaction in the synthesis of the peptidoglycan cell wall. Rollin Hotchkiss had established the cell membrane as another major site of antibiotic action. However, the streptomycin problem that I took up proved to be premature, because this antibiotic was known to block protein synthesis, and nothing was yet known about how to study protein synthesis.

Meanwhile, Dubos had another, indirect influence on my research, which steered it in a new direction, also related to chemotherapy. Organizing a group of authors to produce a textbook of medical bacteriology, *Bacterial and Mycotic Infections of Man*, he invited me to write the chapter on chemotherapy. In doing so I learned that the lysis of bacterial cells by penicillin requires their growth. That fact, and my latent interest in auxotrophic mutants of bacteria, came together in the realization that penicillin should be useful for selecting such mutants, because in minimal medium it should kill the growing wild-type cells, while the mutants, unable to grow in such a medium, should survive (and could be recovered by removing the penicillin and providing the needed growth factor). With this method I soon collected a large number of mutants. Over the next decade, with the generous approval of my chief in the Tuberculosis Control Division of the USPHS, Carroll Palmer, I concentrated on using this material to dissect biosynthetic pathways, especially the long pathway to the aromatic metabolites (7).

As a matter of some historical interest, I might note that Lederberg and Norton Zinder developed precisely the same penicillin method for isolating mutants, at the same time (8). Lederberg, whom I had not yet met, visited my laboratory, and after showing me a short paper that he had recently mailed to the *Journal of Biological Chemistry* he offered to ask the journal to hold it up if I were willing to write a parallel one immediately. I gladly did so, but the journal rejected both manuscripts on grounds of insufficient biochemical interest. In response we decided to publish in the *Journal of the American Chemical Society* (9, 10) rather than in a bacteriological journal (where the papers logically belonged). Moreover, at his suggestion we arranged to have both one-page reprints placed in a single cover. I never felt that this sharing of credit for a simultaneous discovery decreased the credit to either party: science is not a zero-sum game.

I will now return to the mechanism of the lethal action of streptomycin (and the other aminoglycosides). These agents have by far the most complicated action of all antibiotics. The cells remain intact after being killed, and they exhibit changes in the levels of virtually all metabolites; hence there is an enormous, baroque literature on this subject, full of confusing claims for the key effect. In fact, there are several key effects, and I shall briefly outline them here because they were not fitted together coherently until quite recently, more than 40 years after the discovery of streptomycin.

In 1960 Nitya Anand, a visiting scientist from India in my laboratory, discovered that streptomycin treatment of growing cells makes their membrane leaky, as shown by loss of nucleotides and of K^+, and by entry of normally nonpenetrating metabolites (11). Moreover, this membrane damage also allows ready entry of streptomycin itself (12). The damage does not occur if protein synthesis is blocked (as by chloramphenicol), or if the bacterial strain is resistant. We therefore thought that direct damage to a sensitive component of the growing membrane might be the lethal event.

Within a year, however, the membrane damage lost interest, when findings of Spotts and Stanier (13) suggested, as was soon demonstrated, that streptomycin acts directly on the ribosomes of sensitive (but not on those of resistant) cells. Moreover, Gorini and Kataja (14) showed that at sublethal levels the antibiotic causes increased misreading on the ribosome. However, major features of the lethal action were still not understood: whether misreading has anything to do with killing; how action on the ribosome could result in membrane damage; or how the ribosome, which binds tightly only one molecule of streptomycin, could display misreading (in cells) at low antibiotic concentrations but complete blockade of protein synthesis at higher concentrations.

The last question could not be answered until Zinder's discovery of RNA phages, which made available a natural, intact messenger RNA. One could then study the process of initiation of translation, a process that had been artificially bypassed in earlier studies with synthetic polynucleotides. My colleagues Brian Wallace and Phang C. Tai found that when streptomycin binds to an initiating ribosome it causes complete blockade of further synthesis; but when the ribosome is past initiation and engaged in chain elongation, in which the bound ligands make it less flexible, the antibiotic binds in a different way, with a transient, less drastic effect: slowing of synthesis, and misreading (15). It was thus possible to explain how low concentrations (binding primarily to chain-elongating ribosomes) or high concentrations (binding to all ribosomes as they initiated) could have such different effects on cells. Membrane damage remained unexplained.

Which of these actions is responsible for the lethal action on the cell? Spotts and Stanier emphasized, in their influential paper in 1961, that when a drug has multiple actions the art of the investigator is to dissect the key action from the epiphenomena. And that was the goal of all of us for many years. But a few years ago I got a simple idea (which could have arisen 20 years earlier) that connected the effects on the ribosome and on the membrane (16). This link revealed that the lethal action is due not to a single key step but to a series of steps, each of which is equally important.

–≪≪– The highly polar, polycationic streptomycin cannot get into an intact bacterial cell readily, but molecules occasionally enter, perhaps through transient imperfections in the growing membrane or by low affinity for a transport system for some other permeant.

–≪≪– The antibiotic encounters mostly elongating ribosomes and hence causes misreading.

–≪≪– Since all proteins will be randomly misread, some misread proteins will enter the membrane.

–≪≪– The previously missing step is that some of these misread proteins will make the membrane leaky—perhaps because they fit badly into their surroundings or because they are transport proteins, whose distortion by misreading may make their channels excessively large and ungated.

–≪≪– The increased entry of antibiotic through the sites of membrane damage increases the misreading and, hence, causes further damage. This autocatalytic process accounts for the observed rapid transition from impermeability to rapid entry.

-≪- When the cell contains enough antibiotic to saturate the ribosomes all protein synthesis ceases, as a result of blockade of all the ribosomes at initiation sites. Moreover, the process is lethal because the uptake of the highly cationic aminoglycosides (unlike that of reversible inhibitors such as chloramphenicol) is effectively irreversible. (The uptake ultimately yields 100 times as many molecules within the cell as the number of ribosomes, suggesting that the extensive literature on aminoglycoside uptake is concerned with events occurring after the cells have already been killed.)

I think René Dubos would have relished this kind of discovery by his protégé because he loved going beyond simple solutions of problems to discover multiple factors, whether in the pathogenesis of tuberculosis or in the environmental problems that preoccupied him in his later years. The first law of ecology, someone has proposed, is that you can never change only one thing. Similarly, if you poke one part of the cell with streptomycin you trigger a string of phenomena involving multiple other parts.

Let me get back to the comparison of Dubos and Waksman. The obvious lesson is that there is room in science, and need, for many different styles of research. René was gifted at general and philosophical ideas and at paradoxes. But this subtlety has a price. A possible key was suggested to me by a book, unfortunately obscure today, that I picked up in the library of The Rockefeller Institute during my stay there: a set of Silliman Lectures at Yale by the distinguished physical chemist G. N. Lewis called *The Anatomy of Science* (1926). Its arresting first sentence is "The strength of science lies in its naiveté." Waksman was clearly more naive than Dubos in his approach to science, and each was successful in quite a different way.

I would further suggest that Dubos's great influence, on microbiology and later on a wider public, depended much on his intense personality and his flair for dramatizing ideas, as well as on his capacity for recognizing significant ideas. If we had in science people who played a role like that of drama or music or art critics I would say he was a great science critic. His biography of Pasteur shows marvelous capacity to bring out the most significant aspects of each phase of his work, and to make this old history fascinating today. In this connection, I recall Dubos's view (against which I argued) that the personal aspects are of utterly no relevance in presenting the life of a scientist; all that counts, and should interest the audience, are his achievements and his influence.

This view was paralleled by the nature of Dubos's interactions with colleagues, at least so far as I experienced them. What we discussed were always ideas, and not personal matters; and though he had a great influence on my life the relationship remained impersonal, with few contacts. Beneath his showmanship was a great deal of reserve.

The picture that I have been trying to portray has the obvious implication that personality plays a large role in science—more than might be expected of a field whose advance depends, ultimately, on published, objective, verifiable findings. But we use the word *science* with multiple meanings: it refers not only to an objective body of knowledge but also to the activities that aim at adding to that body; and this activity is highly subjective. We expect scientists to assimilate from the literature, and to build on, the findings that are relevant to their interests. And that generally happens, when the contributions are close to what we are already doing. But major shifts in our motivation or attention are likely to come more from personal contacts than from reading. That is why lectures remain so important.

This proposition is vividly illustrated by another episode in the field of chemotherapy. A few years after I left Dubos, Susumu Mitsuhashi, an early postdoctoral fellow in the newly established tuberculosis research laboratory, returned to Japan, and he soon wrote me in great excitement about experiments demonstrating the appearance of multiple drug resistance in one step. I had difficulty understanding his English, and I unfortunately expressed skepticism about a conclusion that seemed to contradict the accepted view: that resistance arises by mutations, each specific for one drug. A bit later a paper by another Japanese researcher, T. Watanabe, appeared in the *Journal of Bacteriology* and described convincingly, in excellent English, the transfer of multiple resistance in one step by a plasmid. Since this paper referred to a number of publications on the subject in Japanese over the past several years, a review of this literature, otherwise inaccessible in the West, would obviously be of exceptional value.

Accordingly, as an editor of *Bacteriological Reviews* I invited Watanabe to write such a review, and it appeared in this widely distributed journal (17). But to my surprise, during the next five years it stimulated no effort to pursue the observations outside Japan, though research funds were readily available at that time. Apparently scientists in the West assumed that this problem, found primarily in *Shigella*, was peculiar to Japan because of the use of human excrement as fertilizer—it couldn't happen here. However, after five years the problem was picked up in this country by a former postdoctoral fellow of mine, David Smith, and by others. Drug resistance plasmids quickly became one of the liveliest areas in microbiology, with major implications for bacterial and molecular genetics and for evolution, as well as for epidemiology and infectious disease. My suspicion is that if Watanabe or Mitsuhashi had been able to give a lecture in the style of

Dubos at a national meeting in this country, the subject would have developed explosively.

All this, of course, is speculative. But I am on more solid ground in emphasizing that an important feature of René Dubos's personality was his power to make you pay attention to what he was saying and to make you think about it. You could hardly forget a conversation that you had with him. And since I have discussed his limitations as well as his virtues, I would like to emphasize that my year with Dubos was by far the most intellectually exciting and inspiring in my scientific career, though I had already studied in several outstanding laboratories before coming to Rockefeller. I am sure this reaction has been shared by many others who came in contact with him. Indeed, while Dubos's first publication on tyrothricin in 1939 probably further encouraged Chain's pursuit of the purification of penicillin, which had begun in 1938, if there had been a personal contact the influence would no doubt have been even stronger!

References

1. Davis, B. D., and R. J. Dubos. 1947. The binding of fatty acids by serum albumin, a protective growth factor in bacteriological media. *Journal of Experimental Medicine.* 86:215.

2. Davis, B. D. 1946. Physiological significance of the binding of molecules by plasma proteins. *American Scientist.* 34:611.

3. Davis, B. D. 1947. The estimation of small amounts of fatty acid in the presence of polyoxyethylene sorbitan partial fatty acid esters ("Tween") and of serum proteins. *Archives of Biochemistry.* 15:351.

4. Dubos, R. J. 1940. The adaptive production of enzymes by bacteria. *Bacteriological Reviews* 4:1.

5. Dubos, R. J. 1950. *Louis Pasteur, Free Lance of Science.* Boston: Little, Brown & Co.

6. Beadle, G. W. 1950. Biochemical genetics. *Chemical Reviews.* 37:15.

7. Davis, B. D. 1954-1955. Biochemical explorations with bacterial mutants. *Harvey Lectures.* 50:230.

8. Lederberg, J., and B. D. Davis. 1987. This week's citation classic. *Current Contents.* 27 August 1987, p. 16.

9. Davis, B. D. 1948. Isolation of biochemically deficient mutants of bacteria by penicillin. *Journal of the American Chemical Society.* 70:4267.

10. Lederberg, J., and N. Zinder. 1948. Concentration of biochemical mutants of bacteria with penicillin. *Journal of the American Chemical Society.* 70:4267.

11. Anand, N., and B. D. Davis. 1960. Damage by streptomycin to the cell membrane of *Escherichia coli. Nature (London).* 185:22.

12. Anand, N., B. D. Davis, and A. K. Armitage. 1960. Uptake of streptomycin by *Escherichia coli. Nature (London).* 185:23.

13. Spotts, C. R., and R. Y. Stanier. 1961. Mechanism of streptomycin action on bacteria: a unitary hypothesis. *Nature (London).* 192:633.

14. Gorini, L., and E. Kataja. 1964. Phenotypic repair by streptomycin of defective genotypes in *E. coli. Proceedings of the National Academy of Sciences of the United States of America.* 51:487.

15. Davis, B. D., P. C. Tai, and B. J. Wallace. 1974. Complex interactions of antibiotics with the ribosome. In *Ribosomes,* edited by M. Nomura, A. Tissieres, and P. Lengyel, p. 771. Cold Spring Harbor, New York: Cold Spring Harbor Laboratory.

16. Davis, B. D. 1987. Mechanism of bactericidal action of aminoglycosides. *Microbiological Reviews.* 51:341.

17. Watanabe, T. 1963. Infectious heredity of multiple drug resistance in bacteria. *Bacteriological Reviews.* 27:187.

FRIEND OF THE GOOD EARTH: RENÉ DUBOS (1901–1982)

Carol L. Moberg

Fifty years ago, microbiologist René Dubos taught the world the principles of finding and producing antibiotics. His discovery of gramicidin in 1939, at The Rockefeller Institute for Medical Research, represents the first systematic research and development of an antibiotic, from its isolation and purification to an analysis of how it cures disease. Gramicidin and its less pure form, tyrothricin, were the first antibiotics to be produced commercially and used clinically. They formed the cornerstone in the antibiotic arsenal and remain in use today.

This remarkable achievement was not Dubos's first, last, or even his most important contribution. To René Dubos, a living organism—microbe, man, society, or earth—could be understood only in the context of the relationships it forms with everything else. This ecologic view led him from investigating problems of soil microbes to those of specific infectious diseases, to social aspects of disease, and, finally, to large environmental issues affecting the whole earth. His fifty-five-year evolution from microbiologist to environmentalist reflects his efforts to build a new philosophy of man's life on earth.

Research Associate, The Rockefeller University. Worked with René Dubos on health and scientific aspects of environmental issues. This essay is reprinted, with permission of The Rockefeller University, from Research Profiles, *summer 1989, number 34.*

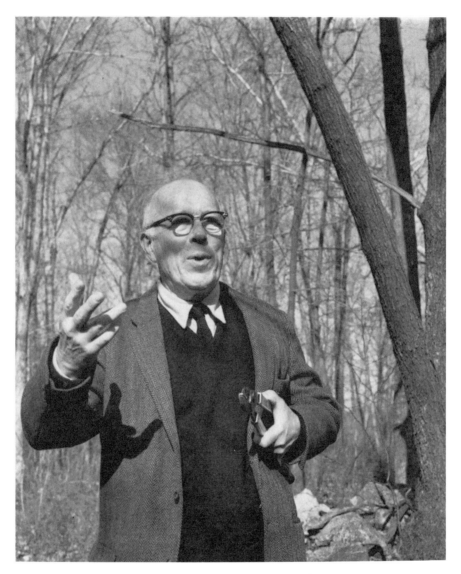

Figure 1. René Dubos, Garrison, New York, 1972. © Lawrence R. Moberg.

Chance Events
and a Prepared Mind

As a child, Dubos lived in small French villages north of Paris where his parents ran a butcher shop. He suffered from rheumatic fever and severe myopia that instilled in him a fear of blindness and a shortened life. Frequently confined to bed, he read avidly and found early heroes in French translations of Buffalo Bill westerns and Nick Carter detective stories. Dubos was inspired to study history when he encountered an essay describing the influences of the Ile-de-France environment on La Fontaine and his fables. These plans were dismissed when his father died in 1919. His mother needed help in the shop, and he suffered another bout of rheumatic fever, preventing him from taking the entrance exam for the Ecole de Physique et Chimie.

On recovering, Dubos passed the exam to the one school still open for enrollment that year. So it was by chance that he attended the Institut National Agronomique to study agricultural science. He excelled in all courses except microbiology. He disliked chemistry and told his mother he would never again enter a laboratory.

After graduation, while writing abstracts for an agricultural journal, Dubos happened to read an article by Serge Winogradsky, a renowned soil bacteriologist. Winogradsky stated that microbes should not be studied in laboratory cultures, but in their natural habitats where environmental conditions and other organisms influence their activities. Dubos embraced this ecological approach to science and decided to study microbiology.

Before resuming his studies, Dubos wanted to visit America. By 1924 he had earned money for passage to the United States on the steamship *Rochambeau*. On board, fate intervened when he met Selman Waksman, the American soil bacteriologist whom Dubos had recently guided around Rome during an international congress on soil science. When Waksman learned Dubos had ambitions but no definite plans to study bacteriology, he offered the young Frenchman a fellowship to study at Rutgers University. Dubos arrived in New York and accompanied Waksman that same evening to the Rutgers campus in New Jersey. Three years later, Dubos earned his doctorate. In the spirit of Winogradsky, Dubos showed that the environmental characteristics of the soil determine which microbes are activated to decompose cellulose, the main ingredient of wood.

In 1927 two more chance events brought Dubos to The Rockefeller Institute (renamed The Rockefeller University in 1965). His application for a National Research Council fellowship was denied because he was not a citizen. The rejection letter contained a handwritten note suggesting he consult with fellow Frenchman Alexis Carrel at Rockefeller. Carrel was kind and considerate but

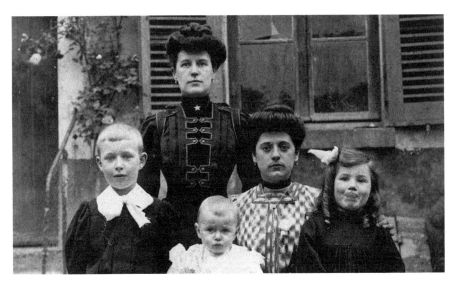

Figure 2. Dubos (left) *with his family at their home in Hénonville, France, around 1908. Courtesy of The Rockefeller University Archives.*

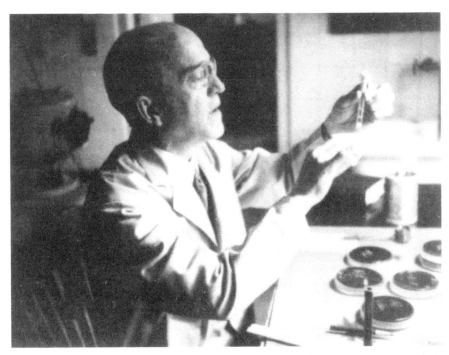

Figure 3. Oswald T. Avery (1877–1955) in his laboratory at the Rockefeller Hospital. Courtesy of The Rockefeller University Archives.

could offer no advice. At lunch, in the now legendary dining room in Welch Hall, Carrel sat the visiting Dubos next to Oswald Avery, whose research expertise with the pneumococcus would lead him to the discovery of DNA as the material of heredity in 1944.

A Plan, Some Patience,
and a Few Pots of Soil

The origin of antibiotics began in Oswald Avery's laboratory at The Rockefeller Institute Hospital, which was trying to produce a therapeutic serum to cure the deadly disease lobar pneumonia. Avery had established that a polysaccharide capsule, or "sugar coat," surrounding the virulent type III pneumococcus bacteria protected it from the body's defense mechanisms. He spent many frustrating years trying to safely decompose this microbe's sugar coat. He knew whoever could find a way to selectively destroy it without side effects would discover a cure for pneumonia. He needed someone in his laboratory to elaborate on what he called his "kitchen chemistry."

Avery brought Dubos back to his laboratory after lunch. He waved a vial of the purified polysaccharide and portrayed the scientific drama that lay within. Dubos replied, rather brashly for a new Ph.D., "Well, I think I can find a microbe to decompose that capsule, and from it I can extract an enzyme." Avery, impressed with this promise, arranged a fellowship for Dubos, little realizing that the problem of the pneumococcus capsules would launch a career that would concern itself someday with the atmospheric capsule enveloping the earth.

In 1975 Dubos recalled his acceptance by Avery. "I don't think there was any other institution in the world then—and perhaps there is none now—that would have taken a person like me, knowing nothing at all about medicine, and coming from an agricultural experiment station, and given him a chance to work in a hospital. It has sensitized me, and ever since I have preached that scientific institutions must remain very flexible and very open."

Within three years, Dubos fulfilled the promise he made to Avery. As a soil microbiologist, he knew organic matter did not accumulate in nature, because countless microbes perform limited, well-defined tasks to recycle this matter. He felt it was a matter of time and patience before he found one specialized in removing the capsule from the type III pneumococcus.

Dubos described the utilitarian 1930s laboratory where he cultivated endless pots of soil in a systematic search for the elusive destroyer. He worked at a wooden desk in a large room that "accommodated a motley assortment of notebooks and simple laboratory instruments—test tube racks, glass Mason jars, droppers for various dyes and chemical reagents, tin cans holding pipettes and platinum loops. . . . The Bunsen burner on each desk served for aseptic transfer of cultures, heat sterilization, preparation of culture media, and also for some chemical operations. We used a great variety of kitchen utensils. . . . [The room had] a few simple incubators, vacuum pumps, and centrifuges . . . [and] a single porcelain sink that served for almost any operation requiring the use of water, from staining slides for microscopic work to preparing extracts of bacterial cultures for immunological tests."

Using a few gardening techniques, he cultivated a soil bacterium from a New Jersey cranberry bog that removed the capsule from the pneumococcus. And, from this bacterium, he isolated an enzyme called the SIII enzyme responsible for the destruction. The triumph came when this enzyme was given to mice infected with pneumonia and it cured them all. Avery was so impressed that he interrupted his summer vacation to verify and publish these findings. The enzyme might have been purified into a therapeutic serum to treat pneumonia in humans, but the sulfa drugs that were just becoming available eclipsed the enzyme's further development. However, Dubos's scientific methods opened the way to gramicidin and the beginning of antibiotics.

A peculiarity of the cranberry bog microbe was that it did not produce the enzyme of its own accord. Dubos discovered the enzyme was produced if the polysaccharide capsule was its only source of food. Once again, he showed the importance of the environment, in this case the soil, in determining which of an organism's multiple potentialities would be manifested. He called this phenomenon "adaptive enzyme," now known as induced enzyme, because enzyme production is an adaptive response to the compelling force of the environment. Dubos considered this his "greatest hour in science," and said it was "one of the most important biological laws I have ever been in contact with."

Dubos had several other successes in finding soil microbes to solve specific biomedical problems. When he decided to look for a soil microbe that could exert broader effects, he used the same cultivation techniques he developed to find the SIII enzyme. This time, however, he tended his soil samples for two years. He wanted to ensure that the only microbe that thrived was one with a cannibalistic appetite for the disease-causing bacteria he was providing as the sole food source to his soil samples. In 1939 Dubos isolated and identified *Bacillus brevis* as the microbe that digested and destroyed other microbes, particularly the pneumococci, staphylococci, and streptococci. From *Bacillus brevis* he extracted the antibacterial agent, or antibiotic, that he named tyrothricin. It contains two polypeptides he called gramicidin and tyrocidine.

Tyrothricin is the partially purified antibiotic whose active ingredient is gramicidin; tyrocidine is ineffective in the body. Within a few months, Dubos and organic chemist Rollin Hotchkiss, a colleague at the Institute, described the bacterial, pharmaceutical, chemical, and clinical aspects of tyrothricin. Although gramicidin proved too toxic to be taken internally, it is highly effective in treating human wounds and other skin infections. Elsie, the famous Borden cow, was stricken with mastitis at the 1939 World's Fair, and was one of the first patients to respond successfully to gramicidin.

Almost immediately, every pharmaceutical company began producing these two antibiotics. Rollin Hotchkiss recalls their 1940 patent application to prevent any restrictions on their production and to ensure their purity: "After an almost hilarious series of negotiations between the unworldly scientists and the worldly lawyers, in which the contents of our notebooks had been translated into thirty-six patent claims, we were called to the business manager's office to assign the patent to the Institute. When we read the clause that ran 'acknowledging the receipt of the sum of one dollar,' we asked if they were serious about the dollar. The business manager, Edric Smith, mumbled something and withdrew, returning a bit later, presumably from the bursar's office, carefully shepherding into the room two half dollars; one for each of us! Dubos, who knew how to make a grand gesture when the time was right, was positively delighted with the evident embarrassment of all concerned." Institute Director Herbert Gasser and Hospital Director Thomas Rivers enthusiastically supported the antibiotic discovery and soon provided the two scientists with new laboratories. The Institute abandoned the patent application in 1943, stating that its objective, to make the discovery freely available to the public, had been achieved.

The work on gramicidin encouraged English scientists Howard Florey and Ernst Chain to revive the dormant research on penicillin that Alexander Fleming found accidentally in 1928. Their article on penicillin's use as a drug appeared in 1940, a year after Dubos's reports on gramicidin. Other scientists began to probe the soil for bacteria that would produce more antibiotics. Dubos's teacher, Selman Waksman, who undertook a search that led to streptomycin, acknowledged that "that gold rush [for antibiotics] should be traced to Dubos's isolation of gramicidin. . . . To obtain the desired results required an analytical mind, an original coordination of all the facts, and especially a new philosophy . . . it was the beginning of an epoch."

Updating the Germ Theory

Even before any of the other antibiotics became available, Dubos predicted bacteria would adapt themselves to these drugs and produce resistant strains. While he recognized great victories in the battle against fatal infections, he warned that these drugs could control, but never conquer, their enemies. In his book, *Mirage of Health* (1959), Dubos compared a "conquer mentality" to the cowboy philosophy in a Buffalo Bill western. "In the crime-ridden frontier town the hero, single-handed, blasts out the desperadoes who were running rampant through the settlement. The story ends on a happy note because it appears that peace has been restored. But the death of the villains does not solve the fundamental problem. The rotten social conditions which had opened the town to the desperadoes will soon allow others to come in, unless something is done to correct the primary source of trouble."

Dubos predicted that increasingly crowded, uniform societies would bring new diseases into being. Eminent scientist, physician, and author Lewis Thomas adds, "Dubos was quite certain that antibiotics in whatever abundance were not going to be the solution. He had a prescient mind and he was especially afraid of what the new viruses might do."

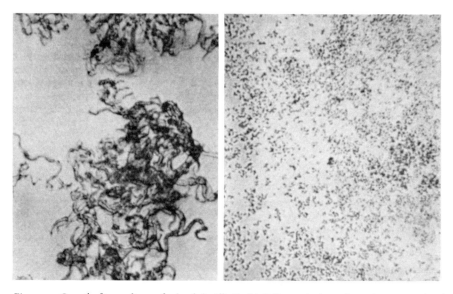

Figure 4. Growth of two cultures of tubercle bacilli. (Left) Cells grow in large clumps in a conventional medium. (Right) Cells show well-dispersed growth in the Dubos-Davis medium. The introduction of nontoxic detergents in the culture medium enabled the first accurate, quantitative studies of various strains of tubercle bacilli and of their disease-causing properties. Courtesy of Vernon Knight, M.D.

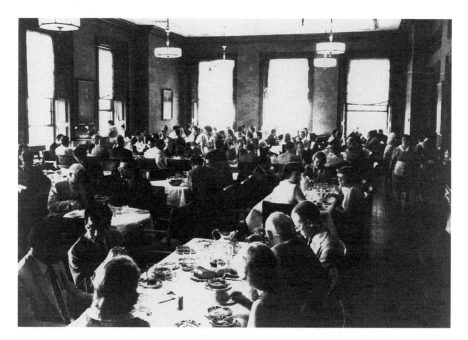

Figure 5. The dining room in Welch Hall, The Rockefeller Institute for Medical Research, mid-1950s. Dubos said, "The dining room where I first met Dr. Avery was the greatest educational institution I have known anywhere. I came to the Institute not knowing a word about medicine. But every day in the dining room at lunch I became slowly sensitized . . . My suspicion is that if it had not been for the dining room at the Rockefeller I would not have been as rapidly successful in science." Courtesy of George Zimbel.

A tragic event in Dubos's personal life turned his interests to the human condition in disease. His first wife died of tuberculosis in 1942, just after he accepted a professorship at Harvard Medical School. Noting that his wife had tuberculosis as a child, he believed it was reactivated by her anguish over family problems in France resulting from the war. Her disease alerted him to the balance between man and bacteria and to the environment's effect on that balance.

After completing wartime studies on dysentery at Harvard, Dubos returned to The Rockefeller Institute in 1944, where he was given complete freedom to establish a laboratory devoted to tuberculosis.

Along with Bernard Davis, Dubos created a culture medium, or special environment, that produces rapid, luxuriant, and well-dispersed growth of tubercle bacilli in the test tube. This advance brought a renaissance in tuberculosis laboratory research. There were also fruitful collaborations with two assistants who returned with him from Harvard. With Cynthia Pierce (now Chase), Dubos pioneered methods for the worldwide standardization of BCG vaccination against tuberculosis, thereby acting on his belief that prevention is better than cure. With Jean Porter, who became his wife in 1946, he co-authored *The White Plague* (1952), a definitive history of tuberculosis as a social disease.

In the 1950s, he and the late James G. Hirsch conducted clinical studies on tuberculosis patients in The Rockefeller Institute Hospital. This group determined that prolonged bed rest, in conjunction with chemotherapy, was not needed and led to the closing of tuberculosis sanatoria, ending an era in medical history. Hirsch recalled how Dubos loved to "play doctor," as he replaced his tan lab coat with a physician's white one and "joined rounds on the ward to visit and show human concern for 'his' patients." This clinical work led to the collaboration of Hirsch and Zanvil A. Cohn, who pursued studies at The Rockefeller University on human defense mechanisms to fight infection and disease. Today, Cohn continues the tradition of the Dubos laboratory by studying the natural reactions of the human body, collectively known as the immune response, that determine the course and outcome of an infection.

Lewis Thomas observes that "although Dubos was not a doctor, he learned more about medicine than most physicians. He knew the power of scientific medicine to reverse mortal infections. But he also knew that mankind's changing of his own environment has much more to do with susceptibility or resistance to infection than anything in the modern pharmacopoeia."

In the 1960s, Dubos investigated the effects of malnutrition, toxins, and stress, and demonstrated how these external factors increased susceptibility to tuberculosis. After The Rockefeller Institute became The Rockefeller University, Dubos's graduate students enlarged his investigations by testing modern environmental influences such as crowding, pesticides, and enzymes in detergents on resistance to other diseases.

Working and thinking ecologically, Dubos's revisions in the germ theory implicated the total environment as a determinant of disease. He showed that a microbe is necessary but not sufficient to cause disease. He reasoned that men coexist with microbes, both good and bad. He found disease-producing microbes are not inherently destructive and can persist in a quiescent state in the body for long periods. The important element in disease, he determined, is not infection but rather any stress that alters resistance, provokes the onslaught of illness, and then determines the outcome of the disease. Dubos's new theme became "if we want to improve our physical and spiritual well-being, we must first understand and then control our impact on our surroundings." For these contributions, infectious disease specialist Walsh McDermott referred to Dubos as "the conscience of modern medicine."

The Conscience
of Human Ecology

To many, Dubos is known as an environmentalist, a scholarly elder statesman, author of some two dozen books, and spokesman for the health of the earth. He saw this new role as an opportunity to address urgent environmental problems that were anticipated by his unfinished laboratory studies. For him, it was the next step in fulfilling the university motto to put science at the service of mankind.

The transition to environmentalist began in the 1950s. As invitations to lecture on environmental aspects of health and disease grew more numerous, he wrote to Rockefeller University President Detlev Bronk explaining his frequent absences from the campus. He expressed profound gratitude for the opportunity and freedom the university had always provided so that he could develop the cultural as well as the scientific aspects of medicine. Bronk's reply encouraged Dubos to continue his "double life in the laboratory and on the frontiers of a changing society." When Dubos's book *So Human an Animal* won the Pulitzer Prize in 1969, he was drawn into the mainstream of the environmental crusade. With amazing resilience and energy between his seventieth and eighty-first years, he devoted all his skills as speaker and author, coupled with his stature as a scientist, to formulate emerging environmental and social issues for an extensive public audience.

Dubos was a visible environmentalist with his charming French accent and avuncular manners. Tall, vigorous, rosy-cheeked, with durable white wisps on a balding head, he radiated a special *joie de vivre*. One was drawn in immediately by his attentive blue eyes filtered through thick glasses, a shy yet broad smile, and beautiful large hands that enthusiastically punctuated every sentence. He coined numerous mottoes to encompass complex issues, among them "Think globally, act locally," which remains a frequently quoted credo of environmental activists.

Dubos changed the ways we think about the environment. He restated ecology as a science that included man and concerned itself with how people live their lives. William Reilly, then president of The Conservation Foundation, and now Environmental Protection Agency administrator, said "Dubos's career began with a critique of environmental abuses and their effects and it concluded with a plea for confident and informed intervention in nature, a belief—heretical in conservation—that 'man can improve upon nature'. . . . Dubos stood for creation."

Not surprisingly, Dubos's favorite landscape represents man's enhancement of nature. He said that walking under the *allées* of trees lining the entrance and the marble walks to the university was an important element of his life. "Morning and

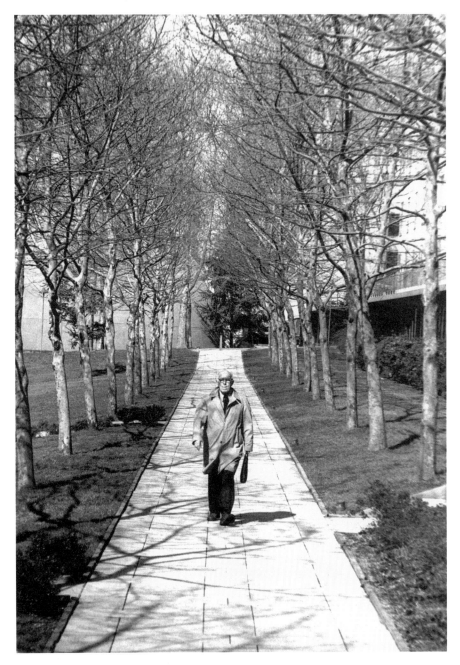

Figure 6. Dubos walking to work under the allées *on the Rockefeller University campus. Courtesy of Medical World News Collection at Harris County Medical Archive, Houston, Texas.*

evening, summer and winter, walking back and forth, I give thanks to those who planted on the grounds of The Rockefeller Institute the rows of sycamore trees which today look so noble against the background of New York City. Always I have in mind the avenue of venerable trees along the roads of France and in the parks where I played as a child." While walking beneath the trees which he watched grow for over half a century, he came to view them as a symbol of the contemplative, peaceful seclusion at The Rockefeller University. "There is no place in the world where I have spent as much time and where I feel more at ease. Whenever I approach the stalwart plane trees of the 66th Street entrance, I know 'this is the place.' "